first place
4health
Bible Study Series

growing in
the fruit of
the Spirit

Published by Gospel Light
Ventura, California, U.S.A.
www.gospellight.com
Printed in the U.S.A.

Caution: The information contained in this book is intended to be solely for
informational and educational purposes. It is assumed that the First Place 4 Health
participant will consult a medical or health professional before beginning this or
any other weight-loss or physical fitness program.

Library of Congress Cataloging-in-Publication Data
Growing in the Fruit of the Spirit.
p. cm. — (First place 4 health Bible study series)
ISBN 978-0-8307-5113-6 (trade paper)
1. Fruit of the Spirit. I. Gospel Light Publications (Firm)
BV4501.3.G78 2009
234'.13—dc22
2009023966

Rights for publishing this book outside the U.S.A. or in non-English
languages are administered by Gospel Light Worldwide, an international
not-for-profit ministry. For additional information, please visit
www.glww.org, email info@glww.org, or write to Gospel Light Worldwide,
1957 Eastman Avenue, Ventura, CA 93003, U.S.A.

contents

foreword

My introduction to Bible study came when I joined First Place in March 1981. I had been attending church since I was a small child, but the extent of my study of the Bible had been reading my Sunday School quarterly on Saturday night. On Sunday morning, I would listen to my Sunday School teacher as she taught God's Word to me. During the worship service, I would listen to our pastor as he taught God's Word to me. Frankly, the idea of digging out the truths of the Bible for myself had never entered my mind.

Perhaps you are right where I was back in 1981. If so, you are in for a blessing you never dreamed possible. As you start studying the truths of the Bible for yourself through the First Place 4 Health Bible studies, you will see God begin to open your understanding of His Word.

Almost every First Place 4 Health member I have talked with about the program says, "The weight loss is wonderful, but the most important thing I have received from my association with First Place 4 Health is learning to study God's Word." The First Place 4 Health Bible studies are designed to be done on a daily basis. As you work through each day's study (which will take 15 to 20 minutes to complete), you will be discovering the deep truths of God's Word. A part of each week's study will also include a Bible memory verse for the week.

There are many in-depth Bible studies on the market. The First Place 4 Health Bible studies are not designed for the purpose of in-depth study, but are designed to be used in conjunction with the rest of the program to bring balance into your life. Our desire is for each member to begin having a personal quiet time with God each day. This time alone with God should include a time of prayer, Bible reading and Bible study. Having a quiet time is a daily discipline that will bring the rich rewards of balance, which is something we all need.

God bless you as you begin this exciting journey toward a balanced life. God will richly bless your efforts to give Him first place in your life. Remember Matthew 6:33: "But seek first his kingdom and his righteousness, and all these things will be given to you as well."

Carole Lewis, First Place 4 Health National Director

introduction

First Place 4 Health is a Christ-centered health program that emphasizes balance in the physical, mental, emotional and spiritual areas of life. The First Place 4 Health program is meant to be a daily process. As we learn to keep Christ first in our lives, we will find that He is the One who satisfies our hunger and our every need.

This Bible study is designed to be used in conjunction with the First Place 4 Health program but can be beneficial for anyone interested in obtaining a balanced lifestyle. The Bible study has been created in a five-day format, with the last two days reserved for reflection on the material studied. Keep in mind that the ultimate goal of studying the Bible is not only for knowledge but also for application and a changed life. Don't feel anxious if you can't seem to find the *correct* answer. Many times, the Word will speak differently to different people, depending on where they are in their walk with God and the season of life they are experiencing. Be prepared to discuss with your fellow First Place 4 Health members what you learned that week through your study.

There are some additional components included with this study that will be helpful as you pursue the goal of giving Christ first place in every area of your life:

- **Group Prayer Request Form:** This form is at the end of each week's study. You can use this to record any special requests that might be given in class.

- **Leader Discussion Guide:** This discussion guide is provided to help the First Place 4 Health leader guide a group through this Bible study. It includes ideas for facilitating a First Place 4 Health class discussion for each week of the Bible study.

- **Two Weeks of Menu Plans with Recipes:** There are 14 days of meals, and all are interchangeable. Each day totals 1,400 to 1,500 calories and includes snacks. Instructions are given for those who need more calories. An accompanying grocery list includes items needed for each week of meals.

- **First Place 4 Health Member Survey:** Fill this out and bring it to your first meeting. This information will help your leader know your interests and talents.

- **Personal Weight and Measurement Record:** Use this form to keep a record of your weight loss. Record any loss or gain on the chart after the weigh-in at each week's meeting.

- **Weekly Prayer Partner Forms:** Fill out this form before class and place it into a basket during the class meeting. After class, you will draw out a prayer request form, and this will be your prayer partner for the week. Try to call or email the person sometime before the next class meeting to encourage that person.

- **Live It Trackers:** Your Live It Tracker is to be completed at home and turned in to your leader at your weekly First Place 4 Health meeting. The Tracker is designed to help you practice mindfulness and stay accountable with regard to your eating and exercise habits. Step-by-step instructions for how to use the Live It Tracker are provided in the *Member's Guide*.

- **Let's Count Our Miles!** A worthy goal we encourage is for you to complete 100 miles of exercise during your 12 weeks in First Place 4 Health. There are many activities listed on pages 255-256 that count toward your goal of 100 miles. When you complete a mile of activity, mark off the box listed on the Hundred Mile Club chart located on the inside of the back cover.

- **Scripture Memory Cards:** These cards have been designed so you can use them while exercising. It is suggested that you punch a hole in the upper left corner and place the cards on a ring. You may want to take the cards in the car or to work so you can practice each week's Scripture memory verse throughout the day.

- **Scripture Memory CD:** All 10 Scripture memory verses have been put to music at an exercise tempo in the CD at the back of this study. Use this CD when exercising or even when you are just driving in your car. The words of Scripture are often easier to memorize when accompanied by music.

welcome to
Growing in the Fruit
of the Spirit

At your first group meeting for this session of First Place 4 Health, you will meet your fellow members, get an overview of your materials and find out what you can expect at weekly meetings. The majority of your class time will be spent learning about the four-sided person concept, the Live It Food Plan, and how change begins from the inside out. You will also have a chance to ask any questions about how to get the most out of First Place 4 Health. If possible, complete the Member Survey on page 205 before your first group meeting. The information that you give will help your leader tailor the next 12 weeks to the needs of the whole group.

Each weekly meeting begins with a weigh-in for members. This will allow you to track your progress over the 12-week session. Your Week One weigh-in/measurement will establish a baseline of comparison so that you can set healthy goals for this session. If you are apprehensive about weighing in every week, talk with your group leader about your concerns. He or she will have some options for you to consider that will make the weigh-in activity encouraging rather than stressful.

The day after your first meeting, begin Week Two of this Bible study. As you open yourself to the truth of Scripture and share your hopes and struggles with the members of your group during the next 12 weeks, you'll find yourself becoming the healthy child of God you are designed to be!

Week Two

growing
in love

SCRIPTURE MEMORY VERSE
But God demonstrates his own love for us in this:
While we were still sinners, Christ died for us.
ROMANS 5:8

A story is told by the early Christian apologist Jerome (AD 347–420) that when the apostle John grew old and frail, his disciples would carry him into the church where he was to give his sermon. There, before the members of the church, he would simply repeat, "Little children, love one another." When some of the members grew tired of this sermon and questioned John as to why he always said the same words, he replied, "Because it is the Lord's command. When only this is done, it is enough."

While it is unknown if this story is completely true, there is no doubt that the apostle John understood the importance of love. John mentions God's love 26 times in his Gospel, almost more than all of the other Gospels combined. He mentions God's love *36 times* in his short letter in 1 John, more than any other book in the entire Bible. And at the end of his Gospel, we see exactly how he wanted to be remembered—as the "disciple whom Jesus loved" (John 21:20).

Love is powerful. In fact, researchers now know that without love and touching, infants can experience a condition known as "failure to thrive." Those who develop this condition simply withdraw from their surroundings and become unable to take in the nutrition they need to help them grow. Loving and being loved are absolutely essential to our wellbeing. The problem is, we look for love in the wrong places. There is only one true source of love, and that is the love that God offers us as a fruit of the Spirit.

This week, we will look at this incredible gift of love and how it should change the way we lead our lives.

GOD, THE AUTHOR OF LOVE

Day 1

Dear God, it is hard to comprehend the depth of Your love for humankind. Help me today to grasp just a piece of what You have done for me. Amen.

As we read in the opening passage of the Bible, "In the beginning God created the heavens and the earth" (Genesis 1:1). He created the universe and this planet, and then He created people and gave them the option of free will. They could obey Him or not—it was their choice. And, as we all know, they chose not to obey God, bringing down a curse on all He had created.

But God did not turn His back on His creation. He sent His only Son to redeem that fallen planet filled with willful people—many of whom today *still* don't care about His great gift to them. Not only did His Son come to earth, but He also died a horrendous death on a Roman cross, and then He rose from the dead so that we could claim eternal life. If that isn't love, then what is?

Today, we will look at a passage from 1 John that explores the nature of God's love.

Read 1 John 4:7-16. What argument does John make for why we should love one another? What does this have to do with the nature of God (see v. 7)?

_____

_____

_____

_____

What does John say about those who do not show love (see v. 8)?

_____

_____

_____

_____

According to John, what did God do to demonstrate His love? What did that enable each of us to do (see v. 9)?

_____

_____

_____

_____

What should our response be to that act of God's love (see v. 11)?

_____

_____

_____

John states that even though we have never seen God, we can know that He lives in us by the way we love others. In what ways are you revealing God in your life by your love for others?

_____

_____

_____

_____

What guarantee does John say we can count on in verse 16? What comfort should this provide to us when things don't go our way and we are tempted to question God's care for us?

_____

_____

_____

_____

"God is love." As you conclude today's study, take a few moments to reflect on this fact and thank Him for the love He has demonstrated in your life.

Dear Father, Your very nature is love. Thank You that You loved me enough to send Your Son to die in my place that I may share in eternal life. Amen.

JESUS, THE FULFILLMENT OF GOD'S LOVE

Day 2

Lord, thank You for Your incredible love for me. Thank You for sending Jesus as the demonstration of that love. Amen.

From the moment Adam and Eve ate the forbidden fruit from the Tree of Life, God began formulating a plan to rescue people from their sin. In Genesis 3:15, He tells the serpent, "I will put enmity between you and the woman, and between your offspring and hers; he will crush your head, and you will strike his heel." Jesus was that offspring who would crush Satan's (the serpent's) head even while he inflicted injury on Jesus. He was the fulfillment of that incredible promise and the ultimate demonstration of God's love.

If we could only begin to grasp a little of what God did for us—the love that He showed us—in giving us His only Son, it would revolutionize our lives. We would still have struggles, but we would approach them with a completely different mindset, knowing that God is truly in charge, understands our need and will be with us along the way. Within us, there would be a deep abiding joy that no circumstances could touch.

Today, we will consider how Jesus' death on the cross was the fulfillment of God's love for humankind and what that means for each of us.

Read 1 John 2:1-6. What does John say Jesus does on our behalf when we make a mistake and fall into sin (see v. 1)?

_____

_____

_____

What do you think it means that Jesus is the "atoning sacrifice" for our sins (see v. 2)?

_____

_____

_____

_____

Under Old Testament Law, when a person sinned, an offering had to be made in order for him or her to atone or "reconcile" with God. To make a sin offering, a person had to bring a male animal without blemish or defect to the priest. He or she would place a hand on the head of the offering, indicating that the person's guilt was being moved to the animal (see Leviticus 1:4). The animal would be killed, and the blood would serve to cover the person's sin and cleanse him or her from sin. In what ways did Christ's death fulfill this role of a sacrifice? In what ways was it different (see v. 2)?

_____

_____

_____

_____

How is God's love made complete in each of us (see v. 5)?

_____

_____

_____

_____

How has knowing that God loved you so much that He sent His Son to die in your place changed your life?

_____

_____

_____

_____

In Ephesians 5:2, Paul writes, "Christ loved us and gave himself up for us as a fragrant offering and sacrifice to God." As you conclude today's session, take a moment to consider the price that God paid for love. Say a prayer of thanksgiving to Him that from the time sin first entered the world, He sought a way for each of us to be reconciled to Him.

Dear God, You tell us that neither death nor life, nor any powers, nor anything else in all creation, will be able to separate us from the love of God (see Romans 8:39). Thank You for this promise and this gift. Amen.

THE LOVE OF CHRIST WITHIN US   Day 3

Dear God, thank You for being my Father. Thank You that Jesus is my brother, friend, example and counselor. Help me to let His love live through me. Amen.

Think back to the illustration of God sending His only Son to this planet to save fallen people from their sins. When we accept God's gift of salvation, we can begin to experience Christ's love not only in us, giving us eternal life, but also being lived out through us. Jesus said, "Whoever finds his life will lose it, and whoever loses his life for my sake will find it" (Matthew 10:39). He then went on to say, "If anyone gives even a cup of cold water to one of these little ones because he is my disciple, I tell you the truth, he will certainly not lose his reward" (Matthew 10:42).

Today, we will look at one final passage in 1 John in which the apostle urges us to put the love of Christ that is within us into action.

Read 1 John 3:15-23. How does John describe a person who hates others? What does he say about that person's character (see v. 15)?

_____

_____

_____

_____

What should we be willing to do for others if we truly love them (see v. 16)? Is this something you could honestly say you would be willing to do for your brothers and sisters in Christ? How about some of those people in your life who are difficult to love?

_____

_____

_____

_____

Of course, we can demonstrate our love for others in more tangible ways. What are some of the practical ways that we show the love of Christ (see vv. 17-18)?

_____

_____

_____

_____

As we read in the Day One study, we know that God lives in us by the way we love others. This is how we know that "we belong to the truth" (v. 19). What reassurance does this give us for those times when our hearts "condemn us" and we find ourselves struggling with doubts?

_____

_____

_____

_____

What two commands does John state we should obey to please God (see v. 23)?

_____

_____

_____

_____

In what ways have you succeeded in obeying these commands? Think of a specific instance where you helped someone and showed him or her the love of Christ. This could be someone in your First Place 4 Health Group, a family member or even a complete stranger.

_____

_____

_____

_____

As you conclude today's study, say a prayer of thanks to God for giving you those opportunities to be His hands and feet in this world, and ask Him to help you find ways to serve Him more by serving others.

Father God, teach me how to let the love of Jesus flow out through my life to others in need. There is so much that needs to be done that it is overwhelming. Show me my place in Your great plan for this world. Amen.

TWO KINDS OF LOVE Day 4

Father God, I want to learn to love as You love. Teach me from Your Word what I need to know to get started. Amen.

There are two Greek words used in the Bible for our one word "love." The first is *phileo*, which means to have a special interest or affection for a person. It is the kind of love exhibited in friendship—what we often refer to as "brotherly love." The word *phileo* implies a strong emotional connection between individuals.

The second Greek word for love is *agape*. *Agape* is the epitome of love. It is the self-sacrificing love that Jesus exhibited when He died for our sins even though He was sinless. To bring it down to something we can better understand, *agape* is the kind of love a mother exhibits when she stays up night after night with a sick child, even though she is exhausted. She gives out of a selfless love. It is an exercise of the will—

a deliberate choice—and is related to obedience and commitment. That's why Jesus can ask us to love our enemies and those who are not particularly lovable. We don't have to feel anything. We just have to obey.

In today's study, we will examine an interesting conversation that took place between Christ and the Peter in which both of these types of love were discussed.

Read John 21:15-19. To set the scene, the risen Jesus had just performed the miracle of the huge catch of fish on the shore of Lake Galilee. He instructed the disciples to bring Him some fish to cook for breakfast and, after they had eaten, He said to Peter, "Simon . . . do you truly love me more than these?" (v. 15). The word used for love here is *agape*, and the "these" most likely refers to the fish. Given this, what was Jesus asking Peter?

_____

_____

_____

_____

Peter responds, "Yes, Lord . . . you know that I love you." The word that Peter uses for love is *phileo*. Using the description given above, what was Peter saying?

_____

_____

_____

_____

Jesus asks the same question again and receives the same answer using the same Greek words for love. Peter was not ready to make the full commitment of *agape* love. Finally, Jesus asks, "Simon . . . do you love [*phileo*] me?" Peter answers, "Lord . . . you know that I love [*phileo*] you"

(v. 17). Where do you think you are in your relationship with God in regard to the kind of love you are giving Him?

_____

_____

_____

_____

What request does Jesus make after this question? What does this reveal about how we should demonstrate love?

_____

_____

_____

_____

How could you move to a deeper level of love for God?

_____

_____

_____

Dear Father, teach me to love You and others as Jesus would love. Help me to learn the kind of love that seeks to give rather than seeks to receive. Finding that kind of love is the way to true happiness and contentment. Amen.

CHARACTERISTICS OF *AGAPE* LOVE — Day 5

Dear God, sometimes it is hard to love the unlovely. Help me to understand Your kind of agape love better so that I can experience it in my life. Amen.

Before we can be willing to demonstrate *agape* love that Jesus calls us to show to others, we first need to explore the characteristics of this type of selfless love. In 1 Corinthians 13:1-13, one of the most famous chapters in the Bible, the apostle Paul provides an excellent primer on ·

exactly what *agape* love looks like. We'll take a closer look at this passage today.

In the first portion of this passage, Paul explains how while we may have other gifts, if we do not have love, they don't count for much. What are some of the gifts we might have that are meaningless if we do not show *agape* love (see vv. 1-3)?

_____

_____

_____

_____

Paul then begins his explanation of what *agape* love is and what it is not. Fill in the missing words that describe *agape* love in the verses 4-8:

Love is _____, love is _____. It does not _____, it does not _____, it is not _____. It is not _____, it is not _____-_____, it is not easily _____, it keeps no _____ __ _____. Love does not delight in _____ but _____ with the _____. It always _____, always _____, always _____, always _____. Love never _____.

Read verse 11. Why do you think Paul inserted a statement on acting like a child right in the middle of a discussion on *agape* love?

_____

_____

_____

_____

Agape love is the result of growth in our Christian life. It takes time, knowledge, prayer and the discipline of the Lord to grow *agape* love in us. As we grow in grace, we advance in our ability to show *agape* love, but we will never reach perfection in this area of our life on this earth.

When does Paul say we will reach the ability to have perfect *agape* love (see v. 12)?

_____

_____

_____

Based on what you have read in this passage, why does Paul claim that love is the greatest gift of God (see v. 13)?

_____

_____

_____

In what ways have you practiced *agape* love in your lifetime?

_____

_____

_____

Dear God, I want to know what it really means to love others. Thank You for first loving me (see 1 John 4:19) so that I can experience that love and know how to share it with others. Amen.

REFLECTION AND APPLICATION

Day
6

Dear Father, I want to put love, a fruit of the Spirit, into action. Strengthen my determination to make a difference in someone's life today by my love. Amen.

All of us want to share God's love with others and be authentic in our relationships. But how well are we really doing this? Today, we will look at some of our relationships and ask ourselves if the kind of love we have is the brotherly love *phileo* or the more self-giving *agape* love. As you do this exercise, think about the places and times when *agape* love is needed to accomplish what God intends for His kingdom.

In the left-hand column below, make a list of the people for whom you have *phileo* love. These are the people in your life who are easy to love because you already have a relationship with them. They could be friends, family, acquaintances or even your fellow First Place 4 Health members. Then, in the right-hand column, indicate how you have shown *phileo* love to them.

People for whom I have *phileo* love	How I have shown *phileo* love to them

Now, make another list of people to whom God is leading you to demonstrate *agape* love. As we mentioned, *agape* love is a more self-sacrificing type of love, so this may include some individuals in your life who are more difficult to love or some people who you do not know well at all.

People whom God is leading me to show *agape* love	What I can do to show *agape* love to these individuals

Now pray over the names on your lists and allow the Holy Spirit to speak to you about how He wants you to love these people.

Father, I want to put Your command to love others into action in my life. Help me to follow through and really make a difference in someone's life. Amen.

REFLECTION AND APPLICATION

Day 7

Dear God, this is where the rubber meets the road. Am I only going to read the words in this study, but do nothing about them? Help me to love others as You love them. Amen.

Prayer has a way of changing events and people. Maybe there are some people in your life who are unlovable, or at least difficult to love. This could be someone you wrote down on your list yesterday. It could be a brother or sister in Christ who consistently offends you. Or it could even be a family member who just seems to be continually at odds with the rest of the family. Whoever it is, know that if you take the matter to God in prayer, He can do a work in that person's life—and in yours—to alter the relationship for the better.

One effective way to remember to pray for such individuals is to create a prayer book. This is basically a journal or even a notebook in which you write down items about that person's life and your relationship that you want to pray over daily. You can even attach a photo of that person if you have one available. Dedicate a page to each person, and then commit to pray for that person for a specified period of time.

It is amazing what can happen when we let love reign in our hearts. We can never know where that love might take us. We can only know that as we give our lives to God and allow Him to guide our actions, our love for others will grow, and God will be honored.

Dear God, today I will embrace the love You have given me and allow it to guide my heart and actions. Thank You for this remarkable gift. Amen.

Group Prayer Requests

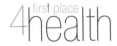

Today's Date: _____

Name	Request

Results

_____

_____

_____

_____

_____

_____

growing in hope

SCRIPTURE MEMORY VERSE

*"For I know the plans I have for you," declares the LORD,
"plans to prosper you and not to harm you,
plans to give you hope and a future."*

JEREMIAH 29:11

Hope in the life of a believer implies more than just having an optimistic belief that events and circumstances will work out for the best. As Christians, God has given us the hope that one day we will be with Him in eternity. For us, this present reality is not all there is, and we can actually look forward to the day when this life is over and we will be reunited with our Father in heaven.

It is that kind of hope that gave the apostles the ability to stand up to any trial that came their way. The apostle Peter, for example, endured a number of persecutions for the sake of Christ. In Acts 5, we read how he and the other apostles were arrested and flogged by the Jewish authorities. Later, in Acts 12, he was arrested by King Herod and thrown into prison.

Yet despite these trials and many others, he could say, "Praise be to the God and Father of our Lord Jesus Christ! In his great mercy he has given us new birth into a living hope through the resurrection of Christ from the dead, and into an inheritance that can never perish" (1 Peter 1:3-4).

God has given each of us the gift of hope. He never intends for us to live in despair, but sometimes we have to persevere in spite of the situations we face so that we can see our hopes realized. As Charles L. Allen once wrote, "When you say a situation or a person is hopeless, you are slamming the door in the face of God." So, let's not be guilty of hopelessness—of slamming the door in God's face. God's hope is abundant, and it is for us.

Day 1 — THE POWER OF HOPE

Dear God, when I am tempted to despair, help me to remember that my hope is in You. You will never abandon me or fail me. Thank You for always being with me. Amen.

All of us face situations in life that cause us to lose hope. But chances are that few of us will ever experience the number of misfortunes that befell a man named Job in the Bible. Job's story is one of the grimmest accounts in Scripture, and yet, despite everything that befell him, time and again Job expressed the hope he had in God.

When the story begins, Job is doing very well. He is a wealthy man who owns thousands of sheep and camels (in addition to smaller numbers of oxen and donkeys) and is blessed with seven sons, three daughters and a large number of servants. He is "the greatest man among all the people of the East" (Job 1:3). But then Satan approaches God and accuses Him of placing a hedge of protection so that nothing could harm Job. Satan says that this is why Job fears Him—because God is protecting him.

So God tells Satan that He will remove His protective hand from Job, and in one fell swoop Job loses everything. He suffers an immediate economic setback when some nearby raiders carry off his oxen and donkeys. Then he is informed that fire has fallen from heaven and consumed his sheep. Next, he learns that some other raiders have taken his camels. The biggest blow, however, is when he discovers that all of his children have died. He had lost his cattle, houses, servants, children—everything.

Read Job 1:20-22. How does Job react to this news?

_____

_____

_____

_____

Does he blame God? What does this say about Job's character?

_____

_____

_____

_____

Satan is not yet finished with Job. Read Job 2:1-10. What does God allow Satan to take away from him next (see vv. 4-6)?

_____

_____

_____

_____

What does Job's wife tell him to do at this point (see v. 9)? Does Job give up hope (see v. 10)?

_____

_____

_____

_____

How does he interpret what is happening to him (see v. 10)?

_____

_____

_____

_____

Perhaps Job's greatest expression of his steadfast hope in God is found in Job 13:15. What does Job say in this verse?

_____

_____

_____

_____

_____

God wants each of us to place our hope in Him. As you conclude today's study, look up the following passages on hope from the book of Psalms. In the right-hand column, write the promise that God is giving to you when you remain steadfast and trust in Him.

Psalm	Promise of God
Psalm 25:3	
Psalm 33:18	
Psalm 33:20	
Psalm 147:11	

Dear God, help me to remember that when I am facing a seemingly hopeless situation, I can always find You in the darkness of my night. Amen.

THE PROMISE OF HOPE

Dear God, even in seemingly hopeless situations, let me never forget the promise of hope that You have given to me. Amen.

If you've ever heard the phrase "hope against hope," you know that it means to want something intensely even though there is little chance you will ever get it. It means believing that something will happen when all the indications say that it won't. When hope is realized in such situations, it is often nothing short of miraculous.

In the book of Genesis, we read about a man named Abram who was clinging to such a hope. God had promised him that he would become the father of many nations, but now he and his wife were now old and still childless. How could he become the father of nations if he couldn't become the father of even one child? Hanging on to this promise must have not only been difficult for him but must have also made him seem ridiculous in the eyes of others. Those who knew him must have thought him a deluded old man.

In Genesis 12, God promised to make Abram into a great nation. But then nothing happened. In Genesis 15:1-6, we see that several years have passed and that Abram is still waiting. Given this, why is Abram's reaction understandable when God says He is Abram's "great reward" (v. 1)?

_____

_____

_____

_____

How does Abram attempt to "nudge" the promise (see v. 3)?

_____

_____

_____

How does God reaffirm His promise to Abram (see vv. 4-5)?

_____

_____

_____

_____

Every so often, God would show up and remind Abram of His promise. Skip ahead a few chapters to Genesis 17:1-8. Abram is now 90 years old. What does God remind him at this point (see v. 2)?

_____

_____

_____

_____

What does God do in verse 5 to forever remind Abram of His intentions?

_____

_____

_____

_____

"Abram" means "exalted father," while "Abraham" means "father of many." This was certainly hope against hope! But what else does God promise Abraham at this time (see v. 8)?

_____

_____

_____

_____

Ten years later, Abraham and Sarah finally see God's promise come true when a son is born (see Genesis 21:1).

Paul sums up Abraham's journey in Romans 4:18: "Against all hope, Abraham in hope believed and so became the father of many nations." Abraham was not in denial about his situation; he knew that his body was as good as dead when it came to procreation. And even if his body could produce a son, he was pretty sure Sarah's never could. But Abraham knew that if God was in this—and he believed God was—the circumstances *didn't matter*. So Abraham went right on believing in the face of impossibility.

As you conclude today's study, think about what you are hoping for today that seems totally impossible. What is it that has become "hope against hope" for you? What do you believe God wants for you in this situation? Can you wait for God's timing?

Dear God, restore to me the gift of hope so I might please You as Abraham did. Help me to commit my situation to You and wait on Your timing. Amen.

OBTAINING HOPE

Day 3

God, You are the source of all hope. Thank You for the hope that You give to me each day and the hope that I have for eternity. You provide all the hope I will ever need. Amen.

What is it that makes tens of thousands of people audition for shows such as *American Idol* each year? Hope. These individuals hope that they have what it takes to make a career in Hollywood. But does hoping for something make it so? Certainly not—it takes talent and a lot of hard work.

In the same way, we can't grow the gift of hope in our lives just by saying, "I'm going to be hopeful." Hope comes through knowing God, the source of hope, and drawing on His strength every day. Hope comes through the work of the Holy Spirit in our lives and through the promises we find in God's Word. Today, we will look at what Scripture says about obtaining hope.

Read Romans 15:4. What does Paul say about the importance of the Word of God in bringing us hope?

_____

_____

_____

_____

In Romans 12:12, he gives us another clue to finding hope. What is it?

_____

_____

_____

Look at Paul's words in Romans 15:13. What encouragement can you find in the prayer Paul prayed for the Roman Christians?

_____

_____

_____

In these verses, Paul provides us with three ways to obtain hope: (1) read the Word of God, (2) be faithful in prayer, and (3) trust in God. Notice also that hope comes to us by the "power of the Holy Spirit." Think about your own life for a moment. Are you feeling hopeless about any situation? If so, what can you do to begin to gain hope?

_____

_____

_____

_____

Read Romans 5:3-5. Why does Paul say that we are to *rejoice* in our sufferings? How does this produce hope in our lives?

_____

_____

_____

Why doesn't hope disappoint us? What is the Holy Spirit's role in this?

_____

_____

_____

_____

As you conclude today's study, think about some of the ways that God has nurtured the gift of hope to you through the power of the Holy Spirit. Say a prayer thanking Him for the promises of Scripture that gives each of us hope.

Dear God, even when things seem hopeless, I want to concentrate on know-ing You better. I know that You can use the tough times in my life to help me persevere, and that through them You can show me hope. Amen.

SHARING HOPE

Day 4

Dear God, there are so many people in my life who need a ray of hope. Help me today to be one who encourages and brings hope to their situation. Thank You, Lord. Amen.

When we're striving to lead a balanced and healthy life, it's easy to lose hope along the way. Losing weight is especially hard. Sometimes it might seem that the numbers aren't moving at all from week to week, and sometimes the numbers even move up instead of down. Likewise, keeping spiritually balanced can be a struggle. Like the number on the scale, it's sometimes hard to see what progress we're making, especially if we feel distant from God on a particular day.

That's why we need encouragers in our life. We need people who can remind us that we "can do everything through him who gives [us] strength" (Philippians 4:13). We need to be reminded that God will give us the strength to do whatever He is asking us to do—including leading a healthy life. If we can grasp this idea, we can also pass on the hope that we have been given.

In yesterday's study, we saw how Paul instructed believers in the Early Church on how they could obtain hope. Today, we will look at how Paul encouraged Timothy, a leader in the church in Ephesus, to remain faithful to the hope he had been given in Christ.

Read 2 Timothy 1:3-11. At the time Paul wrote this letter, he was in prison and had little hope of being released. Yet even though he was in a hopeless situation, he wanted to encourage Timothy to continue his work and lead the church after he was gone. He wanted to share the hope he had found in Christ and remind Timothy to be steadfast in his faith. How does Paul begin this letter (see vv. 3-4)?

_____

_____

_____

After telling Timothy that he longs to see him, what does Paul say about Timothy's faith (see v. 5)?

_____

_____

_____

How does Paul encourage Timothy to be bold in sharing the hope that God has given to him (see vv. 6-7)?

_____

_____

_____

_____

Why do you think Paul asks Timothy not to be "ashamed" to testify about the Lord (see v. 8)?

_____

_____

_____

It's easy to be bold and say we're Christians when we're around people who believe as we do. But it's much harder when we're facing opposition or people are calling us out because of our beliefs. How do Paul's words serve to encourage you and give you hope during such times?

_____

_____

_____

_____

Notice that Paul asks Timothy to join with him in "suffering for the gospel" (v. 8). Why does Paul almost view this as a positive thing? What is the greater hope on which he wants Timothy to focus (see vv. 9-10)?

_____

_____

_____

_____

As you conclude today's study, think about a person in your life who needs hope and encouragement. Make an effort to reach out to that person this week and remind him or her of all the positive things that God has done.

Dear God, let me be quick to encourage others. I know that by strengthening the faith of others, I will be strengthening my own faith. Amen.

ETERNAL HOPE

Day 5

Dear God, thank You for the promise that I will one day live in eternity with You. Thank You for walking through this life with me day by day. Amen.

As believers in Christ, we have been given a gift that far exceeds anything of this world: the hope of eternal life. When Jesus rose from the dead, He made a way for us to be reconciled with God so that we can one day spend eternity with Him. God also has given us the hope of His Holy Spirit while we are on this earth to be our teacher, advocate, companion and friend. When we realize this and focus on this eternal hope that we have in Christ, we can overcome any trial.

Yesterday, we studied how Paul was able to encourage Timothy to be steadfast in his faith even though he knew he would "suffer for the gospel." Paul was able to do this because he knew that Jesus had promised those who follow Him the hope of eternal life. Today, we will look at this hope that Jesus offered.

Read Matthew 5:10-12. What hope does Jesus give to those who remain faithful to Him (see vv. 10-11)?

_____

_____

_____

_____

Why should we be "glad" when we face these difficulties (see v. 12)?

_____

_____

_____

_____

_____

Later, when Jesus is teaching His disciples how to pray, he tells them to address God as "Our Father in heaven" (Matthew 6:9). What hope does our ability to call God our father give us in this life? What hope does it give us in the life to come?

_____

_____

_____

_____

Read John 14:1-4, one of the greatest promises we have been given about our eternal hope in Christ. What does Jesus ask His disciples to do when they are troubled (see v. 1)?

_____

_____

_____

_____

_____

How does Jesus describe heaven? What does He tell the disciples He will do for them (see vv. 2-3)?

_____

_____

_____

_____

_____

If we are believers, and if our faith and knowledge rests on the hope of eternal life (see Titus 1:2), why do you think so many of us live in fear and despair?

_____

_____

_____

_____

_____

As you conclude today's study, take a good look at where your faith is resting. If you are feeling hopeless, how will you change your faith's resting place?

Dear God, it is so easy to get caught up with the temporal things of this world that I lose focus on Your eternal glory. Help me to keep a heavenly perspective and eternal hope with regard to my life here on earth. Amen.

REFLECTION AND APPLICATION

Dear God, sometimes I am less than hopeful, especially about my ability to live a healthier and more balanced live. I can only put my hand in Yours and ask You to give me a hope that is beyond human understanding. Amen.

On this day of reflection, take a moment to review what we've discussed this week on the gift of hope. First, hope has incredible power in our life. It allows us to keep our head up in desperate situations and look to God as the source of our strength. Second, hope provides us with a goal and keeps us moving forward even when circumstances seem impossible. God tells us in His Word how we can obtain hope, and He asks us to encourage others with the hope that we have found in Christ. Finally, as believers, we have been given the hope that we will share eternity with Christ when our time on this earth is complete.

Today, take a personal inventory of the things in your life that bring you hope. In the chart below, form an acrostic from the word "hope" by filling in the things you can be hopeful about that begin with each of the letters.

H	Example: Home
O	Example: Offspring
P	Example: Parents
E	Example: Earnings

If you found yourself feeling hopeless about something as you did this exercise, write a prayer asking God to give you hope in that area.

God, I see the areas in my life where I am trusting You to provide and where I am coming up short. Help me to trust You with my day-to-day life. Amen.

REFLECTION AND APPLICATION Day 7

Dear God, I know that trusting You is a daily activity. Help me take my life one day at a time and one hour at a time and not try to carry my whole life all at once. Thank You, Lord. Amen.

As the Scripture memory verse for this week (Jeremiah 29:11) reveals, God's deepest desire is to give us a hope and a future. He has plans for us that He will reveal as we move forward in our lives. He's not going to give us the whole blueprint at once—that would be overwhelming. Rather, He's going to give us the pieces as we are ready to receive them.

Today, we're going to do something a little different to help reflect on what we've covered this week. Tonight, go outside and look at the stars. Imagine that you are the 90-some-year-old childless Abraham, looking at all those magnificent stars, and you are remembering what God has promised. Your offspring will be like the stars in the sky. You wonder, *How can this be?* Then you hear the small, still voice of God say, "Because I promised it to you."

As you have worked through the study this week, you have had time to consider any areas in your life where you are lacking hope. Now it's time to think about what God has said to you about those areas of your life. What are His plans for you? If you don't know, this would be a good time to ask Him. Seek His will and simply ask Him to reveal His purposes to you.

Dear God, my only hope is in You and in the finished work of the cross. What Jesus accomplished for me on the cross is enough for any need I will ever have. Thank You for filling my life with Your love. Amen.

Group Prayer Requests

4 first place
health

Today's Date: _____

Name	Request

Results

_____

_____

_____

_____

_____

growing in faith

SCRIPTURE MEMORY VERSE

And without faith it is impossible to please God, because anyone who comes to him must believe that he exists and that he rewards those who earnestly seek him.

HEBREWS 11:6

In his book *The 911 Handbook*, Kent Crockett tells the story of how his friend Jeff Patton, an F-15 fighter pilot, was escorting a large formation of fighters in a bomb run during Operation Desert Storm. They were flying in total darkness, which meant that the pilots had to rely completely on their instruments for guidance.

Shortly after crossing into Iraq, Jeff's jet was locked on to by an Iraqi surface-to-air missile. In order to break the lock, Jeff had to violently maneuver his plane. The technique worked, but Jeff soon found he had another problem: the movements had made him dizzy, and he was disoriented. He felt as if the plane were climbing out of a turn, but when he checked his instruments, they told him that he was in a 60-degree dive toward the ground.

At this crucial moment, Jeff had a decision to make: Should he trust his senses or his instruments? Jeff decided to put his faith in his instruments. He rolled the F-15 fighter wings level and pulled the jet upward at seven times the force of gravity. It only took a moment for him to realize he had made the right choice, for when he checked his altimeter, he found he had narrowly cleared the mountains of Iraq by 2,000 feet!

Faith operates much like the instruments of an aircraft. Even though we have never "seen" God, we believe in the Word of God and trust that what it says is true. Even when those around us are trying to convince us otherwise, we know in our hearts that God exists and that He wants to be actively involved in our lives. As the writer of Hebrews puts it, "Faith is being sure of what we hope for and certain of what we do not see" (11:1). This week, we will look at what constitutes faith, where we get it, and what it can do in our lives and in the lives of others.

Day 1 WHAT FAITH IS

Dear God, help me to grasp what faith is all about so I can learn to trust You more. Help my unbelief so that I, in turn, may help others have faith. Amen.

Jesus used the analogy of a seed to describe faith. In Matthew 17:20, He says, "I tell you the truth, if you have faith as small as a mustard seed, you can say to this mountain, 'Move from here to there' and it will move." In the Mediterranean region where Jesus lived, the mustard seed was one of the smallest seeds planted by the farmers. However, with perfect conditions, the mustard plant could grow to a height of 12 to 15 feet—big enough for a bird to build a nest in it.

If we plant our seed of faith and care for it, God will bring life, growth and increase. The harvest that we will receive will be enormous, and we will see marvelous things done for the kingdom of God.

One of the best ways to determine what constitutes faith is to examine incidences in the Bible where Jesus commended people for having faith. In the following table, look up the Scripture in the right-hand column, and then write down the person to whom Jesus was speaking and the commendation He gave.

Scripture	Person	Commendation
Matt. 9:2		
Matt. 9:22		

Scripture	Person	Commendation
Mark 7:29		
Luke 18:24		

Let's look at another incident in which Jesus commended someone for having faith a bit more closely. Read Matthew 8:5-13. What was the centurion's request, and what was Jesus' reply (see vv. 6-7)?

_____

_____

_____

_____

_____

Why did the centurion object to having Jesus come heal his servant? What was his rationale (see vv. 8-9)?

_____

_____

_____

_____

_____

Jesus is astonished at the man's faith and then makes a statement about those who will "take their places at the feast" (v. 11) in the kingdom of heaven. What does Jesus' statement have to do in relation to the faith he has seen in the centurion?

_____

_____

_____

_____

A.B. Simpson once wrote, "True faith drops its letter in the post office box and lets it go. Distrust holds on to a corner of it and wonders that the answer never comes." In what areas of your life are you "holding on" to the letter?

_____

_____

_____

_____

In what areas of your life are you able to "let go" of the letter?

_____

_____

_____

_____

Dear God, help me to have faith even the size of a mustard seed so that You can use it for something great in Your kingdom. Increase my faith, I pray.

Day 2 — WHERE FAITH IS FOUND

Dear God, I admit that sometimes my faith is small. Letting go of control terrifies me. Please show me in Your Word how to trust You more. Amen.

Faith requires us to give up control of our present life to grasp the new life God has for us. We have to give up our hold on all the things that keep us from living the healthy life that God intended before we can embrace that new life. We have to open our lives and risk failure before any real success is possible. Today, we will read about one woman who was willing to take that risk.

Read Luke 8:40-48. When Jesus and His disciples landed on the western shore of the Sea of Galilee, they were met by a crowd of people. Among them was a man named Jairus, who wanted Jesus to heal his daughter, and also a woman who was seeking healing for herself. What does the Bible tell us about her (see v. 43)?

_____

_____

_____

_____

_____

Notice this passage tells us the crowds almost crushed Jesus. In the Greek the word is *sumpnigo,* the same one the Gospel writers use in the parable of the soils to describe the thorns "choking" the wheat and making it unfruitful. Given this, what is surprising about Jesus' question in verse 45?

_____

_____

_____

_____

Notice the woman comes "trembling" (v. 47). She is afraid for her identity to be known. Why was the action she had taken a risk on her part?

_____

_____

_____

_____

_____

According to Jewish Law, the woman's condition made her ceremonially unclean. Those who knew about her condition would have shunned her. But how does Jesus respond (see v. 48)?

_____

_____

_____

_____

Faith grows naturally in the soil of a devoted life. It comes to us by reading, digesting and putting into practice the Word of Christ. Paul writes, "Faith comes from hearing the message, and the message is heard through the word of Christ" (Romans 10:17). Thus, it is when our faith fails that we need to go to the Word of God for encouragement. Look up the Scriptures below and write out the encouragement each verse offers.

1 Corinthians 16:13

_____

_____

_____

Galatians 3:9

_____

_____

_____

Galatians 5:5

_____

_____

_____

Ephesians 3:12

_____

_____

_____

If you find your faith sagging, write out these Scriptures and then pray through them until faith is strengthened in your heart.

Lord, thank You for the assurance that as I put my hand in Yours and walk forward into the future, You will lead me to good things for my life. Amen.

WHAT FAITH CAN DO

*Dear God, I want to accomplish great things for You. Help me
to let go of the control and trust in You completely.
Show me the power of what faith can do today. Amen.*

We need only look to the pages of Scripture to discover the power of
faith. By faith, Noah followed God's instructions to build an ark, and
he and his family were saved. By faith, Abram left his homeland to follow the Lord, and God made him the father of a nation. By faith, Moses
confronted one of the most powerful leaders of his age, and God released the Israelites from oppression. By faith, Peter walked on water,
Paul and Silas rejoiced in prison and were set free, and John wrote down
what the Lord revealed to him in a vision to serve as both a warning and
an encouragement to the Church.

Perhaps one of the most encouraging chapters on faith in the entire Bible is found in Hebrews 11. In this single chapter, we find a ros-
ter of people throughout the ages who had faith and accomplished
great things for God. Today, let's take a closer look at this passage.

In the following table, read the verse from Hebrews 11 listed in the left-
hand column. In the second column, write down the biblical figure
being named, and then write a brief description of why the author of
Hebrews is commending his or her faith.

Verse	Person	Act of faith
Heb. 11:4		
Heb. 11:5		
Heb. 11:7		
Heb. 11:8		

Verse	Person	Act of faith
Heb. 11:20		
Heb. 11:21		
Heb. 11:22		
Heb. 11:23		
Heb. 11:31		

According to verse 13, what was unique about these individuals?

_____

_____

_____

_____

What were these people longing for (see vv. 14-16)? What will be the reward for their faith?

_____

_____

_____

_____

What great promise (and warning) is embedded in verse 6?

_____

_____

_____

_____

What does the author conclude about these people in verse 39? What was it that they "had been promised" but not received?

_____

_____

_____

_____

On a scale of 1 to 10, how would you rate your faith? How can you increase your faith so that you can accomplish great things for God?

_____

_____

_____

As you conclude today's study, consider some of the ways that God might be calling you to "step out in faith." You can do great things for the kingdom of God—but you have to be open to His call!

> *Dear God, thank You for these great examples of faith in the Bible. Help me to be confident in my faith and in the fact that You will always be with me. Thank You, Father. Amen.*

WHY FAITH IS TO BE SHARED Day 4

Lord, I have found a wonderful gift in my faith in You. Help me pass it on to others who do not know You. Help me to continue to grow in faith. Amen.

When we come to Christ, we bring the raggedness of our sinful existence to Him, and He gives us a new robe of righteousness. He lifts us out of our sinful state, cleans us up and makes us shine again. He renews our minds and creates a pure heart within us.

We have been given this incredible gift, but we are not to keep it to ourselves. In Matthew 28:19-20, Jesus told His disciples, "Go and make disciples of all nations, baptizing them in the name of the Father and of the Son and of the Holy Spirit, and teaching them to obey everything I have commanded you." As believers in Christ, we need to share with those in our lives the gift of faith and hope that we have found in Christ. We are to reach out to those who are still dressed in the filthy rags of sin and show them that they can be made clean through the redemption that Christ brings.

Today, we will look at some Scriptures that can help us to share our faith.

Read Romans 3:23. Imagine you are sharing your faith with someone who claims he or she doesn't need God's gift of salvation because he or she is basically a "good person." How can this verse help you show that it isn't enough in God's eyes?

_____

_____

_____

_____

Read Romans 6:23. How can this verse help you show that person the true penalty for his or her sin? What hope can it help you share with that individual?

_____

_____

_____

_____

Read John 3:16. How can this verse help you show another person what it cost God to give each of us the gift of eternal life?

_____

_____

_____

_____

Read John 1:12 and 1 John 1:9. According to these verses, what does the person need to do to escape the penalty for his or her sin? What will be the result?

_____

_____

_____

_____

Read Revelation 3:20. What does Jesus promise to do when the person steps out in faith and accepts Christ as his or her Savior?

_____

_____

_____

_____

There are many more Scriptures for leading another person to faith, but with just these six Scriptures, you have enough (with the Holy Spirit's help) to lead another person to faith in Jesus. So, do you know anyone who has not received God's gift of salvation? Think about how you will share the love of God—and your faith—with him or her this week.

Dear God, help me to look for the lost and have compassion on them. Help me reach them for Your kingdom. Amen.

THE RESULT OF FAITH

Day 5

Dear God, I am so glad I am in Your family. But what is so amazing is that not only do I get to know Your redemption here on earth, but also the joys of eternity to come. Thank You, Father, for the gift of faith. Amen.

Faith gives us the strength to face each day armed with the knowledge that God will be with us every step of the way. It gives us the comfort in knowing that we can call on our heavenly Father when we are in need and that He will provide. It gives us the ultimate hope in knowing that when we leave this earth, we will live with God for all eternity.

Of course, when we are caught up in daily struggles of life, it can be easy to lose sight of this truth. We know that "no mind has conceived what God has prepared for those who love him" (1 Corinthians 2:9), but we don't always live our lives as if we are really experiencing that hope.

The good news is that we're not alone. Even Jesus' closest disciples had questions about eternal life. In Matthew 19:16-22, we read the story of a rich young man who approached Jesus and asked how to obtain everlasting life. When Jesus told him that he had to sell his possessions on earth and give to the poor to get treasure in heaven, he went away sad because he had great wealth. What is interesting is the conversation between Jesus and the disciples that followed. We will look at this today.

Read Matthew 19:23-30. What does Jesus say about the rich young man? What do you think He means by this (see v. 23)?

_____

_____

_____

_____

_____

There have been many interpretations of what Jesus meant when He said, "It is easier for a camel to go through the eye of a needle than for a rich man to enter the kingdom of God" (v. 24). However, they all point to the same general conclusion: Entry into the kingdom of God was difficult for this man who had much because it required him to sacrifice much. Why did this prompt the disciples' next question (see v. 25)?

_____

_____

_____

_____

What incredible promise does Christ reveal in verse 26?

_____

_____

_____

What does Peter ask about the disciples' coming rewards in heaven (see v. 27)? What was it in Jesus' comments about the rich young ruler that prompted this question?

_____

_____

_____

What does Jesus reveal to Peter and to all of us about the future glory that awaits those who are faithful to Him (see vv. 28-29)?

_____

_____

_____

What comfort can we take from these words when we are sometimes anxious about the great unknown beyond death?

_____

_____

_____

_____

Thoughts such as these come to the forefront from time to time, and especially when we have lost a loved one. If you have had such a loss, spend some time thinking about what Jesus said to comfort His disciples. Write a prayer asking for His help in accepting that faith is eternal.

Lord, with You everything is possible. Thank You for providing the means by which I can have eternal life. Help me to not to cling to the things of this world but to focus on Your eternal glory. Amen.

REFLECTION AND APPLICATION

*Father, I am amazed at the part that faith plays in my relationship with You.
Please strengthen my faith from day to day as I learn more about You. Amen.*

Faith doesn't always require a huge step on our part, but it will always
stretch us in some way. Sometimes, faith will require us to step out on
a limb and do something that might seem counterintuitive at the time.
When such moments come they will not be comfortable, but we can
know that God will always use such times to help us grow in our faith
and develop in our relationship with Him.

After Paul's dramatic conversion in Acts 9, during which he was
blinded, God called a man named Ananias to visit Paul in Damascus
and pray for him to restore his sight. At the time, Paul was known as one
of the greatest persecutors of the Church, and Ananias was understand-
ably apprehensive about the request. "Lord," he said, "I have heard many
reports about this man and all the harm he has done to your saints in
Jerusalem. And he has come here with authority from all the chief
priests to arrest all who call on your name" (vv. 13-14).

Following God's instruction would put Ananias's life in jeopardy,
and he wanted to be absolutely certain that this was what God was asking him to do. When God confirmed that is was, Ananias stepped out
in faith and did as the Lord had commanded. Paul's sight was restored,
and he became one the leading figures in the Early Church.

Today, think about some of the ways in which you can stretch your
faith. If you are not already doing so, give to your church, a charitable
organization or some other cause as God leads you. If you are just getting by, this might seem counterintuitive at first, but you will be amazed
at how such a simple act will help your faith to grow. Remember that
God can meet your needs without money being involved. God can meet
your needs with no cash exchanging hands.

*Dear God, today I ask for You to lead me in ways that will stretch my faith.
Help me to learn about Your faithfulness. Help me to give up control. Amen.*

REFLECTION AND APPLICATION

*Dear God, thank You for Your gift of faith and the other fruit
of the Spirit that You have provided to me. Thank You for
helping me to grow in understanding of who You are. Amen.*

When our faith is low, it often helps to pray through some of the promises that we read in God's Word. After all, Scripture is what ultimately builds our faith. So today, think about some of the needs in your life that are causing you to worry and spend some time with God, praying through the following passages.

Lord, You tell me to be strong and courageous. I will not be afraid or terrified, because I know that You, the Lord God, will always be with me. You will never leave me or forsake me (see Deuteronomy 31:6).

Lord, I need Your wisdom. You tell me that if I lack wisdom, I should go to You—the One who gives generously to all without finding fault—and You will give it to me (see James 1:5).

Lord, You say that those who take refuge in You are blessed. Today I give You the glory no matter what I am facing, for those who fear You and seek You will lack no good thing (see Psalm 34:8-10).

God, thank You for the promise that I will not toil in vain or bear children doomed to misfortune. Thank You for Your blessings on me and my household. Before I even call out, You say that You will answer; while I am speaking You will hear (see Isaiah 65:23-24).

Lord, today I will agree with those in my First Place 4 Health group in prayer, for You say that if two people on earth agree about anything they ask for, it will be done by our Father in heaven (see Matthew 18:19).

Group Prayer Requests

4 first place health

Today's Date: _____

Name	Request

Results

_____

_____

_____

_____

_____

_____

growing in goodness

SCRIPTURE MEMORY VERSE
But the fruit of the Spirit is love, joy, peace, patience, kindness, goodness, faithfulness, gentleness and self-control. Against such things there is no law.
GALATIANS 5:22-23

The goodness of God can dramatically change the course of a person's life. One striking example of this can be seen in the life of George Foreman, a former heavyweight boxing champion.

Growing up, George was an angry young man who had a chip on his shoulder. He used this rage to fuel his boxing career. By 1974, he had amassed an amazing record of 40-0 and had more money than he could spend. Yet he still felt empty inside.

In 1974, George traveled to Zaire, where he was defeated by Muhammad Ali. When he later lost a match against Jimmy Young in 1977, he was at the lowest point he had ever been in his life. But it was then that George experienced the goodness of God in a profound way. He let go of all of the anger that he had built up over the years and allowed God to change his heart.

George quit boxing and began preaching the goodness of God to everyone he met. He opened up a youth center in downtown Houston and became an ordained minister of a church. Only the goodness of God could have changed George's life in such a profound way.

No one enjoys difficult times, but it could be that there is no better time to learn about the goodness of God than when things are tough. As the author of Lamentations states, "The LORD is good to those whose hope is in him, to the one who seeks him; it is good to wait quietly for the salvation of the LORD" (Lamentations 3:25-26). This week, we will study how to grow God's gift of goodness in our lives.

Day
1

GOODNESS COMES FROM GOD

Heavenly Father, in a time when nothing is sure, You are good. There has never been a time when You have failed me. Thank You. Amen.

Charles Kingsley, an English university professor, historian and novelist, once said that "goodness is not merely a beautiful thing, but by far the most beautiful thing in the world." Kingsley believed that nothing—not riches, honor, power, pleasure or learning—could ever compare with having goodness in one's life. Even if no one ever noticed that goodness, it was still the best thing for the person.

God displayed His goodness to His people early in the Bible. In Exodus 33, just before He showed His presence to Moses, He said, "I will cause all my goodness to pass in front of you, and I will proclaim my name, the LORD, in your presence. I will have mercy on whom I will have mercy, and I will have compassion on whom I will have compassion" (v. 19). God passed by, and Moses was allowed to see all of His goodness.

Today, we will look at some of the aspects of God's goodness to us.

In the psalms, David speaks of the goodness of God many times. But perhaps there is no lovelier picture of God's goodness than the one he draws in Psalm 23. What good things does David say the Lord does for us in verses 1-3?

_____

_____

_____

_____

_____

The topic of death is scary for anyone. It is the great unknown, which causes us to fear it. Why does David say that he will not be afraid even when he walks through "the valley of the shadow of death" (v. 4)?

_____

_____

_____

_____

_____

If God promises to be with us even in times when we are in mortal peril, it follows that He will be with us in any situation in life. Because of this, we do not need to fear anything. Finish the following sentence:

I will fear no evil even when I . . .

_____

_____

_____

_____

Notice that David refers to the "rod" and the "staff." These were tools of the shepherd. The rod was a stick about a yard long with a knob on one end, while the staff resembled a modern cane, though longer. Shepherds used these tools as both offensive and defensive weapons to protect the sheep. In what way can we find comfort in this idea of both defensive and offensive tools in the hands of our God?

_____

_____

_____

_____

In verse 5, we are told that God prepares a table for us in the presence of our enemies. In ancient times, that would only occur in the king's tent on a battlefield. Think of yourself as being entertained by the King of all kings after His victory over your enemies. What would you say to Him during that event?

_____

_____

_____

_____

_____

Because God is the author of goodness, and because His Holy Spirit is molding us into the image of His Son, it is reasonable to expect goodness to grow in our lives as we progress in our Christian walk. Paul noticed this among the believers in Rome when he wrote, "I myself am convinced, my brothers, that you yourselves are full of goodness, complete in knowledge and competent to instruct one another" (Romans 15:14). As you conclude today's study, think of the ways that goodness, a fruit of the Spirit, has grown in you since you first came to know Christ.

Dear God, help me to believe in Your goodness even if I am in the valley of death, even when everything is going wrong. Because You are good, I can learn to exhibit goodness in my life. Amen.

Day 2 — THE QUALITITES OF GOODNESS

Lord, I want to follow Your command to help those who are in need today. Help me to always take the time to seek ways that I can do good. Amen.

In Deuteronomy 4:9, Moses reminded the Israelites to "be careful, and watch yourselves closely so that you do not forget the things your eyes have seen or let them slip from your heart as long as you live . . . teach them to your children and to their children after them." Because God is good and we are His children—His emissaries on earth—we need to let the fruit of goodness shine through our lives. Today, we will look at a few specific instructions from Jesus on how we can be good to others.

Read Luke 6:27-35. In the following table, list the specific quality of goodness that Jesus is addressing in each of the indicated verses. (Note that some of the verses have more than one quality.)

Verse	Quality of goodness
Luke 6:27	
Luke 6:28	
Luke 6:29	
Luke 6:30	
Luke 6:35	
Luke 6:35	
Luke 6:35	
Luke 6:35	

To most Jews of the time, the Romans were conquerors—the enemy—and thus were to be opposed and hated. The Romans burdened the people with taxes for maintaining law, order and stability and to fund the four legions of soldiers stationed throughout Palestine. Given this, why would Jesus' statement, "Love [*agape*] your enemies, do good to those who hate you" (v. 27), have been so controversial?

_____

_____

_____

_____

Notice that to Jesus, it was not good enough to resist from doing harm to others. What four things does He command His listeners to do in verses 28-29?

_____

_____

_____

_____

Look at Jesus' words again in verse 29: "If someone strikes you on one cheek, turn to him the other also." In the original Greek, the word "cheek" (*siagon*) could be more closely translated "jaw." Jesus is not talking about a slap on the cheek here but a punch in the jaw. What would be the natural reaction to this? What type of heart attitude is Jesus saying that we must adopt?

_____

_____

_____

_____

What three illustrations does Jesus use to show how Christians should surpass those of the world in demonstrating goodness (see vv. 33-35)?

_____

_____

_____

_____

What does Jesus say those who do good will receive from the Father (see v. 35)?

_____

_____

_____

_____

_____

It is difficult to show goodness to those who do not deserve it, but that is exactly what Jesus is advocating in this passage. How can you show goodness to those in your life who do things to purposely bother you?

_____

_____

_____

_____

_____

Dear God, I know that I'm not always good, but I understand how important it is to seek to do what is right. Help me to exhibit qualities of goodness that will make me more like You. Amen.

GOODNESS IN A DARK WORLD

Day 3

Dear God, when I look in the mirror, I want to see someone who has goodness written on his or her face. Teach me Your ways, O Lord. Amen.

These days, it doesn't take much searching to realize that we live in a dark world. The news is filled virtually 24 hours a day with reports of one type of crime or another being committed and the sad effects it has on the victims. Sometimes it all feels so overwhelming, yet often it takes just one spark of goodness to ignite real change.

In the Sermon on the Mount, Jesus speaks about allowing the goodness of God to shine out from our lives and illuminate the dark world around us. Read Matthew 5:13-16. What does Jesus mean when He says that we are "the salt of the earth" (see v. 13)?

_____

_____

_____

_____

_____

Salt gives food flavor. In the same way, if we are true to our calling and exhibit goodness, we make the world a more palatable place. But what happens when we "lose our saltiness" (see v. 13)?

_____

_____

_____

_____

_____

To have any positive effect on this world, we have to maintain our distinctiveness in Christ. Given this, what does Jesus mean when He then says that we are "the light of the world" (v. 14)?

_____

_____

_____

_____

_____

In John 8:12, Jesus describes Himself as the "light of the world." Why would He be using the same term here to describe His disciples?

_____

_____

_____

_____

_____

How does light affects its environment? How are we to likewise affect our environment?

_____

_____

_____

_____

What should be the goal in doing good deeds for others (see v. 16)?

_____

_____

_____

_____

As you conclude today's study, think about some of the ways that you can let your light shine before others so you can bring glory to God.

> *God, the world around me is often a dark place, but I want to stand out and be an example of Christ to others. Help me to lead a life of goodness. Amen.*

THE PATH TO GOODNESS

Day 4

> *Dear God, each day I have a new opportunity to begin again to do good. Teach me today to draw closer to You, to know You better and to show the fruit of the Spirit in my life. Amen.*

In order to grow in goodness, we first need a "map"—the Word of God—so that we know what God considers to be good and how to get there. The living Word of God has power and can revolutionize our attitudes, priorities and outlook on life. Any goodness within us should be a re-flection of Christ, so it is important to study His example in Scripture and seek to follow it. Today, we will examine what the apostle Paul says about how we can grow to be people of goodness.

Read Galatians 5:16-18. If we are living by the Spirit, how will it affect our desires?

_____

_____

_____

_____

What does the sinful nature desire? What does the Spirit desire? Why can't the two coexist (see v. 17)?

_____

_____

_____

_____

Skip ahead a few verses to Galatians 5:24-26. What do we have to clear from our lives to be people of goodness (see v. 24)?

_____

_____

_____

_____

What does it mean to "keep in step with the Spirit" (v. 25)?

_____

_____

_____

_____

What are we to avoid if we want to lead a life of goodness (see v. 26)?

_____

_____

_____

_____

What is your definition of "goodness"? Does it match God's definition? What would you need to do to live such a life?

_____

_____

_____

_____

_____

Lord, cleanse my heart from unrighteousness. Help me to grow in the goodness that comes from You. Make me all I can be for Your kingdom. Amen.

DOING GOOD FOR OTHERS

Day 5

Father, thank You for Your goodness. I don't deserve it, but I am grateful for it. Help me to think of ways that I can demonstrate goodness to others. Amen.

During the recent downturn in the economy, one of the evening news programs invited viewers to send in stories of people who were helping others out during these challenging times. One of the stories was of a South Carolina girl named Katie who grew vegetables in a garden and gave away the food to the hungry. Katie was inspired to begin the project when she grew a 40-pound cabbage and gave it to a local soup kitchen that cooked it up and fed the hungry.

Another story featured volunteers in Boston who helped children learn to read or improve their reading skills through tutoring. There was also a story about a restaurant owner in Michigan who gave away free meals. Instead of handing customers a bill, he simply gave them a note asking them to consider doing something good for others.

When our lives are filled with goodness, we will be compelled to help others. Today, we will look at ways to do good for others.

Read Deuteronomy 10:18-19. What does God do because He is good?

_____

_____

_____

What are we, in turn, to do for others? Why should we be compelled to do this?

_____

_____

_____

_____

While Jesus lived among us on earth, He set a powerful example of doing good. In Matthew 8 alone, we are given 5 different situations in which He ministered to others. In the following table, look up the Scripture in the right-hand column and then write down the person to whom Jesus ministered and the act He performed.

Scripture	Person	Act
Matt. 8:1-4		
Matt. 8:5-13		
Matt. 8:14-15		
Matt. 8:16-17		
Matt. 8:28-34		

Read James 1:27. In this passage, James implies that engaging in religious activities without helping others is worthless. What two things does James state that God looks for in "pure and faultless" religion?

_____

_____

_____

_____

Who do the "orphans and widows" represent today in our world?

_____

_____

_____

_____

Often we think about doing good for others, but we never quite get there because we have no plan of action. So, today, think about what your plan of action might be for getting started on that "good" thing you believe you are called to do.

Lord Jesus, I desire to follow Your command and help the poor, the fallen and the hungry. Help me put a plan in place today for helping others. Amen.

REFLECTION AND APPLICATION

Day
6

God, I give myself to You anew for the work You would have me do. Amen.

In a world lacking in goodness, we can demonstrate the love of Jesus. We can be the salt of the earth and light that shines to a dark world as a beacon of hope. We can be His hands and His feet, going about doing good.

As you have done this week's study, perhaps you have thought you cannot possibly do one more thing. Life is busy, and there are only so many hours in a day. Yet there is one thing you can do to help others—and you can do it while you are going about the routines of your day.

When you are out for a walk, pray for your neighbors. As you pass the houses on your block, pray for the people who live there. Pray that the Holy Spirit will speak to their hearts and draw them to Jesus. If you prefer to do your walking on an indoor treadmill, use the time to pray for needs in the world. Make your exercise time profitable not only for your body but also for your own spirit and the good of the world. Note that God may speak to you as you are doing your prayer walk, so stick a pad and pencil in your pocket before you head out. When you hear God speaking to you, stop and write down what He says.

Someone once said that "goodness is the only investment that never fails." Stock markets rise and fall, but goodness will always be a sure investment. How will you invest your time to do good in this world?

Father God, help me to see doing good as an eternal investment. I want to be a light to this world that points people to You. Amen.

REFLECTION AND APPLICATION

God, someone said that the journey of a thousand miles begins with one step.
Help me today to take the first step toward doing good for others. Amen.

In 2004, Mark Stuart was riding the crest of fame. About a decade before, he and a fellow classmate had formed a Christian rock band called Audio Adrenaline, and over the band's career the group had sold more than 3 million records, released 18 number-one hit singles and won 2 Grammy Awards. Yet for Mark, the success that came with being the lead singer of a rock band wasn't enough.

Growing up, Mark's parents had been missionaries to Haiti. Mark had seen the incredible need in that nation and had a desire to do something to help the people. He was especially concerned about the plight of the many orphans he saw there—approximately 450,000 by some counts. So, on one trip to Haiti, he and his fellow band members decided to stop simply encouraging others to do something and start actively doing something themselves.

The band purchased a plot of land and began to raise funds to build a children's village. Groups of students from the United States came on short-term missions trips to help build the main house and the surrounding structures. Finally, in 2006, the Hands & Feet Children's Village was completed. A staff was hired and trained, and the center began taking in its first orphans.

As we mentioned at the beginning of the study this week, goodness is an outgrowth of a life lived for God. It is a fruit of the Spirit. On a daily basis, we need to put our roots down deeply in Him and allow Him to show us how to grow the fruit of goodness in our lives. We need to be looking for practical ways that we can serve others who are in need in our churches, in our families, in our communities—wherever we happen to be—and be open to the call of God on our lives.

As you conclude this week's study, take some time today to really think about this concept of doing good unto others. Ask God to show you some practical ways to minister to those in your world. And then be bold! Take that first step of faith and allow God to move in your life and change your perceptions.

> *Dear God, I love You and I want to do Your will in this matter. Use me for Your glory. Allow the fruit of Your Spirit, goodness, to grow within me. Thank You, Lord. Amen.*

Group Prayer Requests

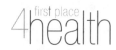

Today's Date: _____

Name	Request

Results

_____

_____

_____

_____

_____

growing
in joy

SCRIPTURE MEMORY VERSE
Do not grieve, for the joy of the LORD is your strength.
NEHEMIAH 8:10

Heller Keller was an American author, activist and lecturer. At the age of nine months, she contracted an illness (possibly scarlet fever or meningitis) that left her deaf and blind. Unable to communicate by either sight or by sound, Helen had to find other ways of communicating with people so that she could understand them.

Over time, Helen's other senses became heightened to compensate for the loss of her sight and hearing. Eventually, she was able to actually sense whether people had joy in their hearts merely by touching their hands. "Those I meet are doubly eloquent to me," she once said. "I have met people so empty of joy that when I clasped their frosty fingertips it seemed as if I were shaking hands with a northeast storm. Others there are whose hands have sunbeams in them so that their grasp warms my heart. It may be only the clinging touch of a child's hand, but there is as much potential sunshine in it for me as there is in a loving glance for others."

We can't hide what we are from many people for very long. What is in our inner life will inevitably spill out to our everyday life. A sincere life—a genuine life—will pour over others and bless them. This week, we will look at this fruit of the Spirit and try to determine how we can spread joy to others.

JOY AND REDEMPTION

*Lord, help me to understand and rejoice in what You have done by
redeeming us, and help me to share that good news with others
so that they may also know the joy of redemption. Amen.*

"Redemption" is a wonderful word because it means something that
has been lost is bought back, atoned for or repurchased. When Adam
and Eve sinned in the Garden of Eden, humankind was separated from
God and the relationship with Him was lost. But then God sent His
Son to redeem us and to restore the relationship. Jesus paid the price
for our sin, bought us back and assured us a place in heaven. We now
belong to God! We are heaven bound! Knowing this should make us
extremely joyful, and we can and should begin to rejoice in our redemption. There are many psalms that are outbursts of joy. Today, we will examine one of these and see how it relates to finding joy in redemption.

Read Psalm 71:1-24. In verses 1-4, the writer acknowledges that there is
wickedness abroad on the earth. What is his plea to God in these verses?

In you, O LORD, I have taken refuge; let me _____ _____ _____ _____
_____. _____ me and _____ me in your righteousness;
_____ _____ _____ to me and _____ me. Be my _____ ____ _____,
to which I can always go; give _____ _____ ___ _____ me, for you
are my rock and my fortress. _____ me, O my God, from the hand of the
wicked, from the grasp of evil and cruel men.

How does the psalmist describe the Lord in verses 5-6? Why does he
state that he will ever praise Him?

_____

_____

_____

_____

_____

In verses 8, 17 and 19, the psalmist lets go with a burst of joy. What does he say?

_____

_____

_____

_____

How does he express his joy to the Lord in verses 22-24?

_____

_____

_____

_____

Why does he say that he will "shout for joy" in verse 23?

_____

_____

_____

_____

THE MESSAGE version of the Bible describes the idea of God being a rock and a fortress as "a guest room where I can retreat." Where do you go when life gets tough? Why do you choose that place?

_____

_____

_____

_____

When the angels came to announce the birth of Jesus to the shepherds, the first thing they said to them was, "Do not be afraid. I bring you good news of great joy that will be for all the people" (Luke 2:10). Look at that phrase again: good news of great joy. Christ came to redeem us, and once He is within us we are to have joy—that deep abiding sense of well-being that circumstances cannot touch.

Dear God, thank You for redeeming me. Forgive the times when I forget all that You paid to redeem me. Help me in those times when I feel depressed and unhappy not to lose my joy. Help me to remember in those times that I belong to You. Amen.

Day 2

WHEN JOY IS GONE

Dear God, I confess that I am not always as joyful as I should be. Help me today to rekindle the joy that can be found in You. Amen.

Take a look around and you will realize that there are unhappy, miserable people in the world—and that some of them are believers. Why is this? Why aren't we all living out the joy that God has placed within us? Why do so many of us need to pray, "Restore to me the joy of my salvation," as David prayed in Psalm 51:12?

Perhaps if we looked at why David prayed this, we could gain some insight as to what was going on in his heart at the time and what might be going on in ours. At the time David wrote this psalm, he had just been caught in a sin. In the spring of that year, when the kings of Israel went to battle with their troops, David decided to stay at home. One night, he got out of bed and walked on the roof of his palace. He looked over at his neighbor's house, and there he saw his neighbor's wife, Bathsheba, bathing. She was beautiful, so he decided he wanted her for his own.

To make a long story short, Bathsheba soon sent word that she was pregnant with his child. David tried to fix the matter first by trying to get Uriah, her husband, to come home from the battlefront and return to his wife, and then by having his commander put Uriah on the front lines, where he would be killed. The second plan worked. But God saw what had happened, and He was very displeased. So He sent the prophet Nathan to confront David about his sin. David realized that he had lost the joy of his salvation—and it was some time before he regained it.

Read Psalm 51:1-19. What is David's first request of the Lord (see v. 1)?

_____

_____

_____

_____

_____

What is his second request (see v. 2)?

_____

_____

_____

_____

What confession does David make to the Lord in verse 4?

_____

_____

_____

_____

After David has confessed his sin, what does he ask of the Lord? In the table below, write out David's requests in verses 7-12:

Psalm	David's request
Ps. 51:7	
Ps. 51:7	

Psalm	David's request
Ps. 51:8	
Ps. 51:8	
Ps. 51:9	
Ps. 51:9	
Ps. 51:10	
Ps. 51:10	
Ps. 51:11	
Ps. 51:12	
Ps. 51:12	

Have you ever been in a situation where you felt you needed God to restore to you the joy of your salvation? What was that situation? What caused your loss of joy? How did you handle that issue?

_____

_____

_____

_____

_____

In verse 16, David says that God does not delight in burnt offerings. What kind of offerings do please God (see v. 17)?

_____

_____

_____

_____

If you have lost the joy of your salvation, in what ways could you make the kind of offering that David talks about in this verse?

_____

_____

_____

_____

Father, it is enough that You love me and have redeemed me. Restore to me today the joy of my salvation, and renew a right spirit within me. Amen.

JOY IN EVERYDAY LIFE | Day 3

Lord, make me an instrument not only of Your peace, but of Your joy. Use me to bring joy to others. Amen.

God created this world for us, and He wants us to take joy in the beauty of His creation and find joy in our fellowship with others. Unfortunately, as we have seen, it can be all too easy to lose that joy. Today, we will look at a church in the New Testament who was experiencing a bit of a joy crisis.

Read Philippians 4:2-7. What was going on among the members of this church (see vv. 2-3)?

_____

_____

_____

_____

How would such a problem have affected the joy of the congregation?

_____

_____

_____

_____

Notice that Paul doesn't scold them for having this problem. What does Paul tell them to do, and how long does he tell them to do it (see v. 4)?

_____

_____

_____

_____

In the *King James Version*, the word "moderation" is used in verse 5 instead of the word "gentleness." How does doing something that brings joy—such as eating—fit in with your goals in First Place 4 Health if it is done in moderation?

_____

_____

_____

_____

How can you stay within the guidelines of healthy eating and still enjoy your food?

_____

_____

_____

_____

What does Paul say the result will be if we trust in God and present our requests to Him (see vv. 6-7)? How should this bring us joy?

_____

_____

_____

_____

God, teach me how to enjoy life—in moderation—and let me be free in sharing that joy with others. Thank You for Your guidance. Amen.

SPREADING THE JOY

Lord, when the shepherds heard the angels' message of joy, they could not wait to share it. Today, let Your love and joy be evident in my life. Amen.

As we mentioned in the introduction to this week, what is in our inner life will inevitably spill out to our everyday life. If we live a life for Christ and experience His joy on a daily basis, that joy will naturally flow out of us and bless others. Today, we will look at how we can always spread joy to others regardless of our circumstances.

Philippians is often referred to as the "epistle of joy" because of its numerous references to joy and rejoicing. What is interesting is that Paul was evidently in prison when he wrote it. Read Philippians 1:12-19. Why was Paul rejoicing in his immediate situation (see vv. 12-13)?

_____

_____

_____

_____

What did Paul say was another positive result of him being in chains (see v. 14)?

_____

_____

_____

_____

Paul goes on to state that some preach the gospel of Christ for less-than-pure motives. Why did even knowing this cause him to rejoice (see vv. 15-18)?

_____

_____

_____

_____

Why does Paul state that he will continue to rejoice, despite his situation (see v. 19)?

_____

_____

_____

_____

Even when our circumstances are bleak, we can find things in which to rejoice. Bring this teaching into your life today. In what ways are you following Paul's example?

_____

_____

_____

_____

In which areas are you failing? How could you change the way you are living with regard to spreading joy?

_____

_____

_____

_____

Dear God, take control of my life so that everyone knows the King is in residence in my life. Let others know when I touch them to help that there is the sunshine of Your love in my hands—in me. Amen.

Day
5

JOY THAT LASTS

*Dear God, let me take all the pieces of what I have learned about joy,
a fruit of the Spirit, and put them into active practice in my life. Amen.*

Martin Lloyd-Jones, a successful preacher in the 1920s and 1930s in England, once wrote the following about joy: "The Scriptures tells us that we should always rejoice. Take the lyrical Epistle of Paul to the Philippians, where he says, 'Rejoice in the Lord always, and again I say rejoice.' Happiness is something within ourselves; rejoicing is in the Lord." We have a *choice* as to whether we will be joyful or not. Whatever happens, we can *choose* to be joyful about our circumstances. When we do this, we will have a joy that lasts in our lives.

There are more than 242 references to the word "joy" in the *New International Version* of the Bible. Each verse is an inspiration for us to remember God loves us and that His love is eternal. Begin today's session by looking up the following verses, and then write down the phrase from each that refers to joy.

Psalm 5:11

_____

_____

_____

Psalm 30:11-12

_____

_____

_____

Psalm 50:23

_____

_____

_____

Psalm 90:14

_____

_____

_____

1 Thessalonians 5:16-18

_____

_____

_____

Using these verses, write down several ideas about how you can deliberately rejoice each day in your own life.

_____

_____

_____

_____

In Psalm 4:7, the psalmist writes the following about God's joy: "You have filled my heart with greater joy than when their grain and new wine abound." The Israelites, like many of the other cultures in the region, depended on a good harvest to sustain their lives. List some of the good things God has brought into your life that are like an abundant harvest.

_____

_____

_____

_____

In what ways do these gifts from God bring you joy?

_____

_____

_____

_____

As you are thinking about these, remember that God's plan is for us to be joyful both now and forever. That's why He sent Jesus to be our Savior.

Dear God, I am looking forward to spending eternity in heaven with You and knowing all the joy You will provide. Amen.

REFLECTION AND APPLICATION

Dear God, joy is a wonderful fruit of the Holy Spirit. Thank You for making it available to me. Please continue to help me always rejoice in You. Amen.

Praying through passages of Scripture is a wonderful way to experience joy. So, today, try praying through one particular passage of Scripture: Psalm 126. This is a wonderful psalm to pray whenever you are feeling low and need a fresh infusion of the joy of the Lord in your life. You can follow the prayers given below or write out a prayer of your own based on this passage in your prayer journal.

Lord, You fill our mouths with laughter and our tongues with songs of joy. You have truly done great things for us (see vv. 2-3). Amen.

Lord, as a river in the desert brings life and joy, You will flow over our lives, bringing good things to our parched souls (see v. 4). Amen.

God, I know that if we sow good seeds in prayer—sometimes even with tears—we will reap a rich harvest of joy in seeing our prayers answered (see vv. 5-6). Amen.

Another way to let God's words soak into your life is by memorizing Scripture. The First Place 4 Health program stresses the importance of memorizing the Scripture readings for each week. The reason for this is because as you commit Scripture to memory, it will become a part of your thoughts and actions. This week's memory verse is Nehemiah 8:10. Read this verse over a few times, and then write it from memory in the space below. How will you apply this verse to your life this week?

Day
7 ## REFLECTION AND APPLICATION

Thank You, Lord, for the joy You bring into my life. Help me to appreciate the gift of joy that You have given me and to share it freely with others. Amen.

This week, we studied how joy is a vital fruit of the Spirit that we must have each day in order to be healthy Christians. However, sometimes we lose our joy as the stresses of our lives pound it out of us. Because of this, we must be deliberate in our pursuit of joy, which means taking time to reflect on what God has given us. So today, take a moment to be deliberate in identifying all of the blessings that God has bestowed upon you. In the space below, make a list of at least five things that God has given to you recently that have brought you joy:

1. _____

2. _____

3. _____

4. _____

5. _____

We also looked this week at how we should always remember that we belong to God, even when we face struggles that seem to take our joy away. As the author of Psalm 34:19 states, "A righteous man may have many troubles, but the LORD delivers him from them all." So, in the space below, make a list of five ways that the Lord has recently delivered you from difficulties:

1. _____

2. _____

3. _____

4. _____

5. _____

Now that you have identified some of the recent blessings that God has given to you and some of the ways that He has delivered you from difficult situations, take a few minutes to pray over your lists, thanking God for His provision in each instance.

Someone has said that hindsight is 20/20, which is often a true statement when we look back on our lives and see how God has redeemed us, cared for us and loved us. If ecstatic joy in what God has done for you is missing in your life, ask God to restore this fruit of the Spirit in your life. It is God's intention that we be joyful—for now and for eternity.

Dear God, I will rejoice in all things—even when things don't necessarily go my way. Teach me to have lasting joy in Christ. Amen.

Group Prayer Requests

4 first place
health

Today's Date: _____

Name	Request

Results

_____

_____

_____

_____

_____

_____

growing in
peace

SCRIPTURE MEMORY VERSE
*And the peace of God, which transcends all understanding,
will guard your hearts and your minds in Christ Jesus.*
PHILIPPIANS 4:7

Contrary to popular opinion, "peace" does not mean the absence of strife. When a country is at war, there may be a day or two when there is no fighting or bloodshed, but that does not mean that the country is at peace. We see this often in the conflict in the Middle East. On occasion, the nations involved in the fighting may declare a ceasefire and stop the violence against one another, but no one would consider the region to be "at peace." Likewise, just because we do not have turmoil in our lives does not mean that we are at peace.

The word "imputed" is an old-fashioned accounting term that means something is "attributed to" or "credited to" something else. For the purposes of our study, we could say that peace is "credited" to the account of our lives. Peace is the gift of God—a fruit of the Spirit—and it is added to our lives. As Jesus told His troubled disciples in John 14:27, "Peace I leave with you; my peace I give you. I do not give to you as the world gives. Do not let your hearts be troubled and do not be afraid."

This week's study will be a comfort and an encouragement to all those who long for peace. For as we read in the Bible, Jesus has promised to give us not just the absence of strife but also the addition of His peace to our lives.

LOOKING FOR PEACE

Father God, I come to You seeking peace. Not the faulty, fragile peace the world talks about, and not just the absence of trouble, but Your magnificent, all-encompassing peace that transcends all understanding. Amen.

The word "peace" is listed 247 times in the *New International Version* of the Bible. We can surmise from this that anything mentioned that many times is obviously important. Our search for lasting peace begins when we realize that we can't find it on our own and that we must turn to God to receive it.

Begin today's study by looking up the verses in the left-hand column of the following table, and then write an insight about where you might find peace in the right-hand column.

Verse	Where you might find peace
Ps. 29:11	
Isa. 26:3	
John 16:33	
Rom. 15:13	

What overwhelming truth comes to your mind when you read these verses about the source of peace?

_____

_____

_____

_____

Jesus taught about the source of peace. What promise did He make to His disciples in John 14:27?

_____

_____

_____

_____

If Jesus is the source of peace, why do you think people search in so many other places for it?

_____

_____

_____

_____

Where have you been searching for peace? How successful have you been at finding it?

_____

_____

_____

_____

Dear Lord, let me pray with the ancient writers, "The LORD bless you and keep you; the LORD make his face shine upon you and be gracious to you; the LORD turn his face toward you and give you peace" (Numbers 6:24-26).

PEACE WRECKERS

Day 2

Dear God, thank You that You free me from feelings of guilt. I know that guilt is not from You and that it prevents me from experiencing Your peace. Help me to experience Your peace in my life today. Amen.

Many of us make choices from time to time that wreck our peace. In some cases, we choose to eat what we want and then feel guilty about the choice we made. The same goes for exercise. We decide it's too cold or we have sore knees or any number of other excuses for not doing what we know would be best for our body. And we wreck our own peace. Today, let's look at some peace wreckers in the Bible.

Lack of trust is one peace wrecker. Read Isaiah 26:3. What does this verse suggest is the answer to this peace wrecker?

_____

_____

_____

_____

Disobedience is another peace wrecker. Read Isaiah 48:18. What is the peacewrecker talked about in this verse?

_____

_____

_____

_____

If the person to whom Isaiah spoke in this verse had followed God's commands, what would have been the result?

_____

_____

_____

_____

Another peace wrecker that stalks us constantly is *fear*. What is the antidote to fear as described in Psalm 3:8?

_____

_____

_____

_____

One of the most beloved psalms in the Bible is Psalm 23. Yet even in this comforting psalm, we see the issue of fear being addressed in verse 4. Why do you think the psalmist says we don't have to fear evil even though we walk through the valley of the shadow of death?

_____

_____

_____

_____

Facing our fears and thinking about what would happen if they actually came true can help defuse our fear and bring peace. What are you afraid of? What is the worst thing that could happen if what you fear actually occurred?

_____

_____

_____

_____

A serious *illness*—either our own or that of a family member or good friend—can be a peace wrecker. We just can't seem to turn off the worry-machine that swirls in our heads when someone is ill. Read Luke 8:43-48. What was the illness of the woman in this story (see v. 43)?

_____

_____

_____

_____

Besides healing her physical illness, what else did Jesus offer the woman (see v. 48)?

_____

_____

_____

_____

When a peace wrecker comes your way, there is not much you can do but put your trust in Jesus. How will knowing that God promises His peace in all circumstances help you to overcome these peace wreckers?

_____

_____

_____

_____

Father God, I need the power of the Holy Spirit at work in my life to help me in difficult times. May the fruit of the Spirit, peace, shine forth in my life even in the most difficult of times. Amen.

Day 3

MAKING PEACE WITH OTHERS

Dear God, there are some people who just destroy my peace every time I have to interact with them. But I know that You love them, so please help me in this area of my life. Amen.

Because peace is a fruit of the Spirit that resides in us when we become believers, we are able, by the Spirit's help, to make peace with others in the family of God. Of course, this is not to say this will always be easy. Debate, disagreement and even dissension are often a part of life.

Even the apostle Paul had disagreements with the disciples and other leaders in the Early Church. In Galatians 2:11, he writes, "When Peter came to Antioch, I opposed him to his face." The book of Acts tells us that he also had a disagreement with Barnabas about taking John Mark on a missionary trip with them. "Barnabas wanted to take John, also called Mark, with them, but Paul did not think it wise to take him because he had deserted them in Pamphylia and had not continued with them in the work" (Acts 15:37-38). The two had such a sharp disagreement that they parted company, with Barnabas taking John Mark and Paul choosing a new traveling companion, Silas.

Even though we and other believers may have differing opinions at times, we need to remember that we can call upon the Holy Spirit and

His gift of peace during such times. He will guide us into a peaceful solution of our disagreements, even if—like Paul and Barnabas—it means parting ways for a while.

Read Philippians 4:2-3. In this passage, Paul refers to two women who were squabbling in the church. What was Paul's plea to these women?

_____

_____

_____

_____

Who else does Paul encourage to become involved in this dispute? How are they to be involved?

_____

_____

_____

In what ways do you think this faction might have disturbed the peace of the Philippian church?

_____

_____

_____

Perhaps you have been involved in a group (maybe even a First Place 4 Health group!) where two or more members were in disagreement. What did you do to resolve the situation?

_____

_____

_____

_____

The Bible has some specific instructions on how to maintain and restore peace in the Body of Christ. Read the following verses in the left-hand column, and then write down the instruction for restoring peace in the right-hand column.

Verse	Instructions for restoring peace
Lev. 19:18	
Gal. 5:13	
Eph. 4:2	
Col. 3:14	
Jas. 1:19	
1 Pet. 2:17	
1 Pet. 3:8	
1 Pet. 4:8	

Remember that Jesus said, "By this all men will know that you are my disciples, if you love one another" (John 13:35). The ground floor of any peaceful relationship with other believers is love.

Dear God, help me to remember to turn to You in the heat of the moment when I want to lash out in anger at another person. Give me peace within myself and help me to pass this peace on to others. Amen.

MAKING PEACE WITH YOURSELF

*Dear Lord, I may be able to forgive others for wrongs done,
but forgiving myself is another matter. Teach me how to let go of the past,
as I know I cannot live in true peace until I have forgiven myself. Amen.*

A counselor once told a client that when she forgave someone, she cut one of the strings the other person could use to cause her to respond negatively to that individual's actions. It was like cutting the strings on a puppet—the other person could no longer pull the strings and get her to react. When we forgive ourselves, we cut the strings that bind us to the past and are set free. We no longer need to react when others try to draw us into a dispute. However, forgiving ourselves is often a lot harder than forgiving another person. But in order to truly live in the peace that passes understanding, we have to learn to forgive ourselves and make peace with our lives.

The prophet Isaiah expressed a sentiment that many of us feel when we stand in the presence of God either in prayer or in a moment of revelation of our unworthiness. Read Isaiah 6:1-8. What did the prophet say that might also be our prayer in a moment of understanding our human condition (see v. 5)?

_____

_____

_____

_____

_____

What caused him to view himself this way (see vv. 1-4)?

_____

_____

_____

_____

_____

When a seraph (a celestial being) flew to Isaiah with a live coal, what words of encouragement did the seraph offer to him (see vv. 6-7)?

_____

_____

_____

_____

After this event, Isaiah came to peace within himself and he responded in a very different way to God's call. What did he say (see v. 8)?

_____

_____

_____

_____

Think about the apostle Paul and the life he lived before meeting Christ on the Damascus Road. If ever there were a man to despise his past and have difficulty forgiving himself for what he had done to Christians, that man would have been Paul. Yet somehow he managed to accept the complete forgiveness of Jesus and radically turn about to a new life. Read Ephesians 1:4-5. How does Paul say that Christ considers us in His sight?

_____

_____

_____

_____

Read Ephesians 1:18-19. What was Paul's prayer for the believers?

_____

_____

_____

_____

If God has forgiven our past sinful offenses, who are we to continue dragging them around with us? As you conclude today's study, consider whether you have been guilty of carrying around a gunnysack of your past sins and hurts. If so, what will you do today to work to rid yourself of this unnecessary burden that drains life from you?

Father, thank You for Your provision of peace that comes from forgiving myself. Help me every time I am tempted to take up that guilt again. Amen.

PRAYING FOR PEACE

Day 5

Dear God, let there be peace on earth and, if possible, let it begin in me. Let me share the peace that You have put in my heart with others today. Thank You, Lord. Amen.

In 1516, Sir Thomas More coined the word "Utopia" to describe an ideal place in which everyone gets along and there is perfect peace. Unfortunately, because of the fall of mankind in the Garden of Eden and the entrance of sin into this world, there has never been a Utopia on earth. Yet the Bible still gives us instructions to pray for peace on the earth and to especially seek peace and unity among believers. Today, we will look at several passages in which we are commanded to pray for such peace.

In Jeremiah 29:7, we read, "Seek the peace and prosperity of the city to which I have carried you into exile. Pray to the LORD for it, because if it prospers, you too will prosper." Why are we to seek the peace and prosperity of our cities?

_____

_____

_____

_____

Read Ephesians 2:14-22. In this passage, Paul is specifically addressing the issue of breaking down the barriers in the Ephesian church that separated those believers who came from Jewish backgrounds and those who came from Gentile backgrounds. According to Paul, what does Christ desire for these two separate groups of people (see vv. 14-15)?

_____

_____

_____

_____

What is the end result of Christ putting to death hostility and bringing peace to the believers through His sacrifice (see vv. 15-16)?

_____

_____

_____

_____

Paul says that Christ preached peace to those who "were far away" (the Gentiles) and those "who were near" (the Jews). As a result, how were the believers to consider each other (see v. 19)?

_____

_____

_____

_____

_____

In verse 22, Paul writes, "In him you too are being built together to become a dwelling in which God lives by his Spirit." Paul was saying that we are all part of the building that Jesus is constructing on this earth. How do you think praying for peace and seeking reconciliation would make the construction of this building move forward more smoothly?

_____

_____

_____

_____

In another Scripture, Paul writes, "Let the peace of Christ rule in your hearts, since as members of one body you were called to peace" (Colossians 3:15). If you are having a problem letting the peace of Christ rule your heart in any way, what might be the solution?

_____

_____

_____

_____

As you conclude today's study, remember that while there is no Utopia on earth, we can work to get along with each other and bring peace to our fellowships. We can also pray for peace in our home, our church, our community and our country. Let's do that right now.

Dear Father, I pray for the peace of my home, my church, my city and my country. You are the source of everything. I ask that You give to us what we cannot make for ourselves: peace. Amen.

REFLECTION AND APPLICATION

Day 6

Lord Jesus, You said, "Blessed are the peacemakers, for they will be called sons of God." Today, I yield control of my life to You so that I can be used by You to bring peace to my relationships. Amen.

If we have the Holy Spirit living within us, our task is to get to know God and His Son, Jesus, in a personal way. Our task is also to get to know His Word and to put His instructions into action in our lives. It is the Holy Spirit's task to plant the seeds and grow fruit in our lives, and if we have done our part, He will.

In the same way that a tree standing in an orchard cannot "will" itself to bear fruit, we cannot bear fruit in our lives simply by willing it or wishing it. For a tree to bear fruit, it has to receive nourishment through its roots so that it can bloom and grow. One of the fruit of the Spirit is peace, and for that to grow in our lives, we have to allow the Holy Spirit to work in our lives. If we truly seek God, in time we will be overwhelmed with the fruit of His peace.

Here are some promises of God with regard to our peace:

"Great peace have they who love your law, and nothing can make them stumble" (Psalm 119:165).

"You will keep him in perfect peace, whose mind is steadfast, because he trusts in you" (Isaiah 26:3).

"Peace I leave with you; my peace I give you. I do not give to you as the world gives. Do not let your hearts be troubled and do not be afraid" (John 14:27).

To live a balanced life emotionally, physically, mentally and spiritually, we need the peace of God. As you conclude today's session, write a short prayer in your prayer journal in which you confess any lack of peace in your life. Ask God to bring His gift of peace, "which transcends all understanding" (Philippians 4:7), to you regardless of the circumstances.

Lord, let me walk in the strong faith that the Holy Spirit is at work in my life and that He will grow the fruit of peace in me as I continue to seek God in prayer and learn about Him through His Word. Amen.

Day
7

REFLECTION AND APPLICATION

Dear God, You are the source of all peace. Help me to turn to You for peace in my life on a daily basis and in any and every situation. Amen.

The hardest part of learning anything is putting it into practice in our lives on a daily basis. It is so easy to quickly forget what we have learned. We need to remember that God's peace is an antidote to all the turmoil we experience in life. We just need to come to Him and draw on Him as our source of peace.

The Gospel of Mark tells about a stressful situation the disciples were facing. After the miracle of the feeding of the 5,000, Jesus sent the disciples on across the lake while He went to pray. When evening came, He saw the disciples straining at the oars, because the wind had risen. So He went out to them, walking on the lake. Then Mark tells us that "He was about to pass by them" (6:48). Now, why would He do *that*? Why wouldn't He just stop the storm and walk over to the boat? Was He waiting for them to call out to Him? The Bible doesn't say for sure, but what is clear is that when the disciples *did* call out, He immediately said, "Take courage! It is I. Don't be afraid" (v. 51). Then He climbed into the boat with them, and the wind died down.

To help you remember what God wants to do for you in regard to keeping the fruit of peace in your life, make a list of the things that take away your peace in the left-hand column of the following table. Then, to the right of each item, note how remembering what you've learned about God's peace might help you react in the future.

Things that take away my peace	How I will react because of God's peace

Dear Father, when times get scary in the future, help me to remember all that I've learned about You as the source of all peace. Amen.

Group Prayer Requests

4 first place
health

Today's Date: _____

Name	Request

Results

_____

_____

_____

_____

_____

growing in patience

"Patience" is the ability to wait for something, even when it might be difficult to do so. "Perseverance" is sticking to a task and attempting to accomplish it in a determined way, despite any obstacles that might appear or hindrances that might get in the way. Could it be that without patience, perseverance would never happen? Could it also be that perseverance is the mother of patience?

We sometimes read the Bible as if everything in it happened in a matter of weeks, months or years. The truth, however, is that there might have been a lifetime between the time that God promised something to a person and the time that He chose to answer that promise. It is as if we are seeing "mountaintops" of miracles. When we stand on one mountaintop and look across the span of history we may see only the miracles, but if we look more closely, we will see the long valleys of time between those miracles. We may even see the deserts and wilderness that God's people had to pass through before they reached the miracle.

Both patience and perseverance are virtues that we need to grow in our lives. This week, we will read about some people in Scripture who were required to exhibit these traits to see what we can learn from their particular example.

PATIENCE MEANS WAITING

Dear God, sometimes patience isn't one of my better virtues. I want
everything to happen right now or very soon. Help me this week to
learn to have more patience. Amen.

Like us, the people in the Bible struggled with being patient and often
grew weary of waiting on God's timing. As we studied in Week Three,
one of the most notorious examples of this is seen in the story of Abraham and Sarah. God had promised Abraham a son, but it took years and
years for that promise to be fulfilled. And in the meantime, Abraham
and Sarah got tired of waiting and tried to force the will of God. Today,
we'll take a closer look at this story as it relates to having patience.

Read Genesis 16:1-4. What did Sarah do that flew in the face of God's
promise (see vv. 1-2)?

_____

_____

_____

_____

What was Abraham's response? What was the result (see vv. 2-4)?

_____

_____

_____

_____

Once Hagar became pregnant, things began to go wrong quickly. What
did Hagar begin to do? Who did Sarah blame for this change in events
(see vv. 4-6)?

_____

_____

_____

_____

Abraham quickly retreated from the situation and put Sarah in control. What did she do? What was the result (see v. 6)?

_____

_____

_____

_____

This was a mess that could have been avoided if Sarah and Abraham had just had patience and waited on God's timing. They were under the mistaken idea that they needed to "nudge" God's plan along. Who are some other characters in Scripture that you can think of who tried to get ahead of God's plan? (Hint: see Exodus 32:1-4; Numbers 20:7-12; 1 Samuel 13:1-13.)

_____

_____

_____

_____

Patience requires us to trust in God and have faith that He will do as He has promised. So, how are you doing in this area? Do you have times when patience is difficult for you? In the space below, write out some situations in which you struggle with having patience. Pray over each of these and ask God to give you patience in these areas.

_____

_____

_____

_____

Dear God, every day is a new day in learning patience. Let me not grow weary in doing Your will. Let me pass the test of patience today. Amen.

THE PATH TO PATIENCE

Lord, patience is hard. Often, I'm not even sure if I want to go through what it takes to learn it. But I know I need more of it in my life. Please help me to rely on the Holy Spirit for guidance. Amen.

In yesterday's study, we read about the negative consequences of trying to rush God's timing. Clearly, patience is something that each of us needs more of in our lives. It is so easy to grow tired of waiting on the Lord and be tempted to try to move things along through our own efforts. So, how do we grow in patience?

We have mentioned this before, but it is important to remember that the fruit of the Spirit is a natural outgrowth of a life firmly rooted in Jesus Christ and nurtured by the Word of God and prayer. Patience, like many of the other gifts of the Spirit, requires a dependence on God and a belief that He always has the best plan for our lives. It means remaining steadfast when a situation comes our way that tempts us to rush ahead. Often, it takes some trial and error until we get it right.

Have you noticed that oftentimes people who are older and have had more life experiences tend to have a great deal of patience in the face of difficulty? A clue to this can be found in Proverbs 19:11. What is one quality that grows patience?

_____

_____

_____

_____

_____

What does Ecclesiastes 7:8 say about patience?

_____

_____

_____

_____

What does patience have to do with pride? What do we do when we attempt to take the control of our lives from God and rush His timing?

_____

_____

_____

_____

_____

How can learning humility and complete dependence on the Lord lead to greater patience (and less anxiety) in our lives?

_____

_____

_____

_____

_____

In Colossians 1:9-12, Paul gives a list of the things that he had been praying the Colossian Christians would receive from God. List each of these requests below:

We have not stopped praying for you and asking God to _____ ___ _____ the

_____ of his _____ through all _____ _____

and _____ (v. 9).

And we pray this in order that you may _____ a _____ _____ of the

_____ and may _____ him __ _____ _____: bearing _____ in

every _____ _____, growing in the _____

___ _____ (v. 10),

being _____ with all _____ according to his _____

_____ so that you may ____ _____ _____ and _____,

and joyfully _____ _____ to the _____, who has qualified you to

share in the inheritance of the saints in the kingdom of light (vv. 11-12).

In what ways are you willing to open your life to the Holy Spirit so that He can teach you patience—even if it means you will struggle and perhaps have to suffer to learn the lesson?

_____

_____

_____

_____

Patience is an area in our lives in which most of us can grow. As you conclude today's session, write a short prayer asking God to help you grow in patience.

_____

_____

_____

_____

Dear God, patience is often learned in the midst of struggle. Help me not to be discouraged by this, but rather to seek You and learn to rely on Your strength when I am tempted to move ahead too fast. Amen.

Day 3 · PATIENCE AND PERSEVERANCE

Dear God, no one likes trials and troubles—and I'm not volunteering for more than my share—but I know sometimes it takes challenging situations to grow my patience. Help me to rely on You in every situation. Amen.

Anyone who has ever raised a child knows all about the "terrible twos." This is the period of time in children's lives when they begin to be aware of what they want but are unable to communicate this need to their parents or are unable to obtain it for themselves. As a result, they often get frustrated and act out in their anger.

It's a trying time for any parent. Part of the problem is that there is no reasoning with two-year-olds. They want what they want, and there is no logic that parents can present that will convince them otherwise.

With two-year-olds, the parents' "no" just has to be the final word on the matter. No reason can be given until the child matures and can understand their parents' rationale for not giving in to the request. Fortunately, children *do* grow in understanding rather quickly and turn into real little people with whom their parents can have a somewhat logical conversation.

Perhaps this is how God views us when He is trying to teach us patience. We can be willful and stubborn at times and so confident that we are right that God can't get through to reason with us. It is only by going through tough experiences and often reaping the consequences of what we have sown that we can come to understand who God is and who we are. This builds patience and perseverance in our lives. We'll look at this more closely today.

Read James 1:2-3. Why would James consider trials of many kinds "pure joy"?

_____

_____

_____

_____

According to James, what is the purpose of developing perseverance?

_____

_____

_____

Read Romans 5:3-4. How does this passage affirm the idea that we must go through some periods of suffering to learn perseverance?

_____

_____

_____

_____

What does Paul say is the end result of us growing in perseverance?

_____

_____

_____

Read Hebrews 10:32-36. What types of situations had the Early Christians experienced (see vv. 32-34)?

_____

_____

_____

_____

How did they react when confronted with suffering?

_____

_____

_____

_____

What will be the result of their perseverance (see v. 36)?

_____

_____

_____

_____

In what ways can you consider the struggles you may be experiencing as steppingstones to growing the fruit of patience in your life?

_____

_____

_____

_____

Dear God, I want to look at the trials in my life as a means of growing faith and perseverance. Continue to grow patience in me. Amen.

BIBLICAL ROLE MODELS OF PATIENCE

Dear God, I want to learn from the example of others
how to be patient and kind. Show me the places in
my life where I need to change. Amen.

Day
4

In Week Three, we looked at the story of Job and examined how he was able to maintain his hope in the Lord in spite of the horrible circumstances he was confronting. To maintain this hope required great patience and endurance on his part. In fact, his example is so striking that when we speak of someone who is patient, we often state that he or she "has the patience of Job." Yet Job is not the only person in the Bible from whom we can learn the benefits of having patience. Today, we will look at a three other famous figures in Scripture and see how they persevered in their situations.

First, we will look at the story of Noah. The Bible says that Noah was "blameless." Noah was a righteous man who walked with God and obeyed His commands. Read Genesis 6:5-18. What was the spiritual condition of people at the time when Noah started building the ark (see v. 5)?

_____

_____

_____

_____

_____

In what ways would Noah have exhibited patience in order to build a boat of the proportions given in verses 14-16?

_____

_____

_____

_____

_____

Jacob is another biblical character from whom we can learn a lesson about patience. After demonstrating his impatience and claiming his brother's inheritance for himself, he was forced to flee for his life. Later, he met a beautiful young woman named Rachel in the place where he had fled. Suddenly, Jacob had lots of patience. Read Genesis 29:16-27. What did Jacob agree to do in return for Rachel's hand in marriage (see v. 18)?

_____

_____

_____

_____

How did his father-in-law reward his patience and hard work (see v. 23)?

_____

_____

_____

_____

How did Jacob show even more patience after he had been conned by his father-in-law (see vv. 26-27)?

_____

_____

_____

_____

_____

The prophet Samuel also exhibited a tremendous amount of patience with the people of Israel when they whined and begged for a king. At the time, the nation of Israel was a theocracy, with God at its head.

Samuel knew that an earthly king would only bring them troubles. Read 1 Samuel 8:4-21. What did the elders of Israel ask for (see v. 4)?

_____

_____

_____

_____

When Samuel talked with God about this request, what was God's answer (see vv. 7-9)?

_____

_____

_____

_____

_____

Samuel did what God said and warned the people, but it did not change their minds. How did Samuel demonstrate great patience with the people throughout this situation?

_____

_____

_____

_____

_____

Waiting is probably the hardest thing God asks us to do. Often it seems He is a "just-in-time" God, and we don't understand why it has to be that way. We need to encourage ourselves that He has our best interests at heart and wait patiently for Him to change our circumstances.

Dear God, at times I'm guilty of being impatient. Help me to learn from these role models and exhibit more patience in my life. Amen.

LEARNING PATIENCE

Dear God, let me grow in patience day by day. Show me practical ways to be patient with my friends, my family, my work associates and myself. Amen.

Someone once said, "It takes patience to learn patience." The logic of that statement might seem a bit circular in nature, but in a way it is true: it takes time and effort to learn how to wait. We can get into the habit of responding with impatience to anything over which we have lost control. If that includes an outburst of anger, it could lead to us feeling embarrassed and remorseful about the way we reacted. In many ways, learning patience can help us live a less stressful life.

But how can we learn patience? Today, we will look at ways to acquire and grow in this fruit of the Spirit.

The key to patience seems to be in learning what we can control and what we have to submit to God and let Him control. Read Psalm 37:3-6. What three items of instruction does the psalmist give here?

_____

_____

_____

_____

_____

How would trusting in the Lord, delighting in Him and committing our ways to Him help us to have patience in our lives when situations may not be going our way?

_____

_____

_____

_____

_____

How would it help us to have more patience with others?

_____

_____

_____

_____

This passage seems to be telling us to give God control of those things that we cannot control and just take one day at a time. How do Jesus' words in Matthew 6:34 reinforce this idea of living one day at a time?

_____

_____

_____

_____

What comes to mind when you read Matthew 6:34? Does taking one day at a time come naturally to you, or do you find it to be a bit of a struggle? How could living this way lead to greater patience in life?

_____

_____

_____

_____

Learning to have patience with ourselves may be one of the toughest lessons to learn. However, we need to accept that we are humans who are growing, learning and changing all the time. In Philippians 1:6, Paul writes, "He who began a good work in you will carry it on to completion until the day of Christ Jesus." How can this verse help when you are feeling impatient with yourself?

_____

_____

_____

In Luke 5:17-26, Jesus healed a paralytic man and told him that his sins were forgiven. That is what He says to us when we come to Him. So, today, if you have been beating yourself up about a struggle that you have not yet overcome—whether this relates to losing weight or some other issue—realize that He wants you to accept His forgiveness and move forward.

Don't let impatience with yourself hamper the work that God is doing in your life to mature you into the person He created you to be.

Dear God, I need to remember that You are at work in me and that You are not finished with me yet. Thank You for Your patience with me as I learn to live in a patient way. Amen.

Day 6 REFLECTION AND APPLICATION

Dear God, patience truly is a fruit of the Spirit. Thank You for this gift in my life. Today, I ask that You help me move into a new level of patience. Amen.

Here is an idea that requires some courage, but one that has rich rewards if you go through with it.

Get together with one or two friends in your First Place 4 Health group and talk about situations in which each of you gets frustrated and tends to lose patience. This could be impatience with a friend, a family member, a coworker, a fellow churchgoer or even the bank teller who always puts that little sign up right before you step up to the window.

Once you have discussed the situation, do a short role-play. Have one person play the individual who makes you lose patience and try to figure out a different way to react to the situation. After you've done the role-play and have determined what it is about the person or the situation that makes you lose patience, complete the sentences listed below.

I noticed that I began to lose patience when . . .

_____

_____

_____

_____

When I lost patience, I experienced emotions such as . . .

_____

_____

_____

_____

I think what was at the bottom of my feelings of impatience was . . .

_____

_____

_____

_____

When my friends and I discussed ways to avoid becoming impatient in this situation, the best idea for overcoming my impatience was . . .

_____

_____

_____

_____

God, please help me in the future to . . .

_____

_____

_____

_____

*Dear God, thank You for always being patient with me. Help me
to remember that when I lose my patience with others. Amen.*

REFLECTION AND APPLICATION

*Dear God, it is so easy for me to become impatient with my efforts
to take care of my body and achieve a healthy weight. Please help me
this week to have patience, particularly with myself. Amen.*

This week, we've looked at several examples of people in Scripture who developed patience. It's important to note that some of them were required to be patient for long periods of time. To put this in perspective, consider the following:

- Abraham and Sarah waited 25 years for the birth of Isaac (see Genesis 12:4; 17:17)

- Joseph languished for many years in prison before God vindicated him (see Genesis 40:1)

- Moses waited 40 years in the desert to receive God's call (see Acts 7:23)

- Paul spent at least 3 years in Arabia before he began the ministry to which God had called him (see Galatians 1:18-18)

Each of these people waited years before they saw what we would consider results in their lives. This must have taken incredible patience.

Losing weight and living a healthy and balanced lifestyle is undoubtedly one of the toughest areas in which to learn patience. We want to see the pounds fall off, or we want to feel that we have reached a certain point in our spiritual walk with God, and it can be so hard to be patient and not get exasperated with our progress (or lack of it).

Losing weight can be especially frustrating if we've experienced good results in the beginning but over time our weight loss has slowed. We might have even said to ourselves, *Oh, what's the use. I might as well eat what I want. I'm not losing weight anyway.* That's the problem with impatience: it can lead us to sabotage everything we've accomplished so far. Next comes the guilt, the disgust with ourselves, the despair that nothing will ever change—and down and down we spiral.

During these agonizing times of waiting, it can help to read the encouraging promises of God's care and concern for us found in the Bible, such as in 1 Peter 5:7: "Cast all your anxiety on him because he cares for you." As we've mentioned, memorizing each week's key verse of Scripture will help you to call these up at a moment's notice when you are tempted to lose patience and give up. The Word of God can strengthen you when you are feeling weak and encourage you to stay on course.

May God bless you this week as you put your life into His hands and seek to be patient with His plans, patient with yourself, and patient with others.

Father God, thank You for loving even the most impatient of Your children. I want to be a patient and giving person in my home, at work, with friends and in every other place. I know that as I focus on patience, a fruit of the Spirit, You will grow that fruit in me. Amen.

Group Prayer Requests

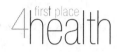

Today's Date: _____

Name	Request

Results

_____

_____

_____

_____

_____

_____

growing in compassion

SCRIPTURE MEMORY VERSE
Therefore, as God's chosen people, holy and dearly loved, clothe yourselves with compassion, kindness, humility, gentleness and patience.
COLOSSIANS 3:12

He had no idea when he loaded up his donkey and set out on his journey that he was walking into the pages of history. He was of a despised race of people and tried as much as possible to stay away from those who hated him so much. He traveled alone, and quickly—it was the best way to avoid the bandits that attacked travelers along the road. Those evil thieves thought nothing of stealing everything a man had, including the clothes he was wearing, and then beating him until he was near death. Yes, better to travel quickly and get off the road before nightfall.

He walked along, urging the donkey forward . . . and then he saw him. There, lying almost on the road, was a man, naked and bloodied and unconscious. What could he do? He had to hurry on . . . but how could he leave another human being just lying there? He stopped, scratched his head and thought for a moment, and then he knew what he must do. He crossed the road and went to the fallen man.

Good, the man was breathing. He poured some water from the skin that was tied to the donkey. The man opened his swollen eyes, saw the cup of water, and parted his parched lips to let the water trickle in. The traveler reached for the oil and wine, and using his own tunic he began tearing strips of cloth to bind up the man's wounds. After a few minutes, the victim began to rouse a little.

"Ah, good, you are conscious," said the traveler. "Do you think you can bear for me to lift you onto my donkey? I need to get you to an inn where you can receive care." With the injured man groaning and moaning, the traveler lifted the man's bruised and broken body onto his donkey. Then he turned and started back toward an inn he had just passed. There, this poor unfortunate man could find help.

Before long, they arrived at the inn and were met by the innkeeper and his wife. The two were appalled by this poor man's condition. "Of course," they said, "We will take him in." The traveler handed the innkeeper two silver coins. "I will pay any extra expense for his care when I return," he said.

Jesus told this parable of the Good Samaritan's act of compassion in Luke 10:30-36. This week, we will explore what compassion really is and how we should exhibit it in our lives as a fruit of the Spirit.

Day 1 — UNDERSTANDING COMPASSION

Dear Lord, I know I cannot practice compassion unless I understand what it means. Teach me today how to be a compassionate person.

Before we can really understand how to exhibit compassion in our lives, we first need to grasp what that term means. The word "compassion" comes from two Latin words, "com" and "pati." *Com* means "together," while *pati* means "to suffer." Thus, a compassionate person is one who suffers alongside another. Some synonyms for "compassion" include benevolence, charity, empathy, grace, kindness, mercy and tenderness. Today, we will look at what the Bible has to say about compassion.

Read 2 Corinthians 1:3-7. How does Paul describe God the Father (see v. 3)? Why do you think He chooses to describe God this way?

_____

_____

_____

_____

According to this passage, for what reason does God comfort us in all of our troubles (see v. 4)?

_____

_____

_____

_____

What does Paul imply that we will share with Christ in verse 5? What else will we be given?

_____

_____

_____

_____

Paul says that there is a reason why he and others who ministered to those in the Corinthian church were willing to be in distress. What was the reason he gives for their willingness to suffer (see v. 6-7; see also 4:15)?

_____

_____

_____

_____

To fully understand what compassion is, we need to look at some of the words that are the opposite. Some of these include "cruelty," "hatred," "indifference," "mercilessness" and "tyranny." Think about some of your actions in the past week. How are you doing in this area of compassion?

_____

_____

_____

_____

Dear God, let me grow in understanding of what compassion truly is so that I can practice it more freely in my life. Amen.

Day
2
THE COMPASSION OF THE FATHER

Lord, I come to You, knowing You have a tender heart toward me. Your forgiveness is always available. Thank You for this gift of compassion. Amen.

Each philosophical tradition has its own view of compassion. In the Jewish tradition, God is seen as the Father of compassion. He exhibits the emotion of a parent for his child. As the prophet Isaiah wrote, "Can a mother forget the baby at her breast and have no compassion on the child she has borne? Though she may forget, I will not forget you! See, I have engraved you on the palms of my hands" (Isaiah 49:15-16). In the New Testament Christian tradition, God is seen as the the "Father of compassion and the God of all comfort" (2 Corinthians 1:3). Today, we will look at this aspect of God the comforter and explore what it can teach us about understanding compassion.

Read Psalm 103:8-18. How does the psalmist portray the Lord in verse 8?

_____

_____

_____

_____

Because God is compassionate toward us, what does the psalmist say He will not do (see vv. 9-10)?

_____

_____

_____

What is the extent of God's love for us? What has He done with our sins (see vv. 11-12)?

_____

_____

_____

_____

How does the fatherhood of God affect His relationship with us, His children (see vv. 13-14)?

_____

_____

_____

_____

This passage of Scripture tells us that God knows how we are put together and that He understands we will sometimes fail because we are human. His response to us is compassion. How can we take comfort from this psalm?

_____

_____

_____

_____

What wonderful promise does God extend not only to us but also to the future generations (see vv. 17-18)?

_____

_____

_____

_____

Compare these words with James 1:17. What promise with regard to our future and God's compassion do you find in this verse?

_____

_____

_____

_____

Dear God, thank You for being the Father of compassion. I know that even when I fall short You will be there to lift me up and set me back on course. Thank You for never changing in Your love and compassion for me. Amen.

THE COMPASSION OF GOD'S SON

Dear Jesus, like a tender shepherd, You watch over us with compassion.
Thank You for loving me beyond human comprehension. Help me to learn
from Your example how I can be more compassionate to others. Amen.

Throughout Jesus' ministry on earth, He cared for those who were "outside" of society—the poor, the orphans, the sick. In His Sermon on the Mount, He told the crowds, "Blessed are the meek" (Matthew 5:5). But who were the "meek"? In our modern world, we define the meek as those who lack courage. But in Jesus' times, the meek could be more accurately described as "the poor in spirit." Jesus was saying that those who realize their spiritual poverty are blessed because they understand that they are powerless to save themselves.

Jesus' day-to-day compassion during His time on earth was only the beginning of His demonstration of His great love for us. We truly cannot comprehend the compassion of Jesus when He went to the cross for us. Jesus willingly came to earth for one sole purpose: to sacrifice Himself for our sins. Today, we will look at the compassion of Jesus, our role model for developing this fruit of the Spirit in our lives.

Let's look at some of the acts of compassion Jesus performed throughout His ministry here on earth. In the following table, look up the Scriptures listed in the left-hand column, and then identify the act of compassion that Jesus showed in the right-hand column.

Scripture	Act of compassion
Matt. 9:35-36	
Matt. 20:29-34	
Mark 1:40-42	

Scripture	Act of compassion
John 11:17-36	
John 12:3-7	

Read Matthew 15:29-37. In this story, Jesus had just returned from Tyre and Sidon and had gone up on a mountainside near the Sea of Galilee. While He was there, crowds began to come to Him. What types of people made up this crowd (see v. 30)?

_____

_____

_____

_____

What immediate act of compassion did Jesus demonstrate (see v. 31)?

_____

_____

_____

Notice Jesus' words in verse 32. What was His concern for those who had come to be healed by Him?

_____

_____

_____

_____

How did Jesus meet this need (see vv. 36-37)?

_____

_____

_____

_____

In what ways has Jesus shown compassion to you? In what ways do you need His compassion in your life right now?

_____

_____

_____

_____

At end of John's Gospel, the disciple said, "Jesus did many other things as well. If every one of them were written down, I suppose that even the whole world would not have room for the books that would be written" (John 21:25). Many of those "other things" that Jesus did were acts of compassion. And He is still doing those acts of compassion today.

Dear God, Your mercy and grace are brand new to me every morning. Sometimes we take Your compassion for granted. Help me to remember all that You have done for me. Amen.

Day 4

OUR NEED FOR COMPASSION

God, sometimes I can get so busy that I don't consider the needs of others. Help me to be intentional in how I demonstrate Your compassion. Amen.

Sheep find amazing ways to get into all kinds of trouble. They wander off and get lost. They follow other sheep and end up in places where they shouldn't be. They fall into ditches and can't get out by themselves. They also often fall prey to other predatory animals. Sheep need a compassionate shepherd to take care of them and keep them safe.

We are a lot like these sheep. We find amazing ways to get ourselves into trouble. We wander off from the path that God wants for our lives and end up lost. We follow the crowd and end up where we shouldn't be. We fall and need to be lifted up again and restored. We fall prey to the attacks of the enemy. We are a vulnerable lot, and we need a compassionate Shepherd who will take care of us and keep us safe.

Today, we will look at this analogy of the shepherd and the sheep and examine how each of us needs the compassion of our Savior.

Read John 10:11-18. In this passage, Jesus uses the example of a shepherd to teach about how He shows compassion for us. He refers to Himself as "the good shepherd" who "lays down his life for the sheep" (v. 11). In ancient times, shepherds would lie down across the opening of the sheepfold at night so that no one could steal the sheep. The shepherd would also stay on guard and not let any animal come near the sheep to do harm. What else does Jesus say the good shepherd will do for his sheep (see v. 15)?

_____

_____

_____

_____

_____

What is the attitude of the shepherd's heart in performing this act of compassion (see v. 17)?

_____

_____

_____

_____

If Jesus is the good shepherd and we are to be like Him, what should be our concern for the other sheep of His flock? What should our concern be for "those other sheep that are not of this sheep pen" (v. 16)?

_____

_____

_____

_____

Jesus repeats a phrase throughout this passage. What is that phrase? What does that tell you about the depth of His compassion for us?

_____

_____

_____

_____

In what ways are you like these sheep in need of a good shepherd?

_____

_____

_____

It's amazing when you consider the depth of God's compassion for us. He saw us in our sinful state and knew that the only way we could be saved and restored to relationship with Himself was through the sacrifice of His Son. Jesus is the good shepherd who, as the ultimate act of compassion, lay down His very life for the sake of His sheep.

> *Dear God, I need Your compassion on a daily basis. Allow me to accept that compassion and reach out to others who are also in need of Your grace. Amen.*

Day 5 — COMPASSION FOR OTHERS

Dear God, I love to have compassion extended to me, but sometimes forget to give it to others. Teach me how to grow compassion in my life. Amen.

A few years ago, a successful college professor felt God calling her to the African country of Swaziland to begin a home for orphans. Her thinking was that the children she could rescue would first of all come to know Jesus as their Savior, and then she would see that they were educated in various skills so that they could become the next generation of leadership so desperately needed in the country. At the heart of it all was her tremendous compassion for these children and that land of gentle people.

Compassion sends us to places we never thought we would go. It causes us to do things we never thought we would do. It makes us weep and pray and educate ourselves and sacrifice. Compassion says "yes" to the needs of those around us. And compassion enables us to reach out to those who have been cast out by society and share the goods news of Christ with them. We will look at this type of compassion today.

Read John 4:4-26. In this story, Jesus is sitting at a well in the region known as Samaria when a woman comes to draw water from it. When He asks her for a drink, she is amazed that a Jewish man would ask a Samaritan woman for water, for there was a long history of hatred between the two regions of the country. "How can you ask me for a drink?" she asks. How does Jesus respond (see v. 10)?

_____

_____

_____

_____

The woman is confused by by the term "living water" and asks Jesus to clarify. How does He explain what this "living water" is (see vv. 13-14)?

_____

_____

_____

_____

The woman asks for this water so that she will never thirst again. She is still thinking literally at this point—she is hoping to never have to come to the well again. In response, what does Jesus ask her to do (see v. 16)?

_____

_____

_____

_____

How does the woman answer? How does Jesus then get to the heart of the matter (see vv. 17-18)?

_____

_____

_____

_____

The sin that Jesus exposes in her life was one that often resulted in death by stoning. This woman was an outcast from her society, yet here Jesus was, speaking to her and sharing the good news He had come to bring. Given all of this, in what ways was this encounter between the two an act of compassion on Jesus' part?

_____

_____

_____

_____

If this story had happened to you, what do you think your initial response to what Jesus did—the way that He handled it—would have been?

_____

_____

_____

_____

As you conclude today's study, think about how you can demonstrate compassion to others. Remember this does not always have to be something major—just a simple act of kindness to someone who is hurting and is in need can go a long way in bringing healing to that person's life.

Dear God, teach me Your ways, especially as they relate to having compassion. There is so much need in the world. Help me to be available for your purposes, regardless of whether they are big or small. Amen.

REFLECTION AND APPLICATION

*Dear God, teach me about compassion as a fruit of the Spirit.
Teach me how to exhibit more compassion in my life. Amen.*

Day 6

"Compassion fatigue" is a form of burnout that manifests itself as physical, emotional and spiritual exhaustion. It often occurs in deeply caring people who try to do too much to serve others without giving enough thought to their own needs. Those who suffer with compassion fatigue can develop symptoms such as hopelessness, decrease in joy, stress, anxiety and a negative attitude.

To avoid such fatigue, those who selflessly serve others in this manner have to find time to do something to recharge their batteries every day. They must take the time for self-reflection and identify what's important in their lives. Then they must make a plan for living that includes taking time for what they have deemed important and begin to live in a way that reflects their decisions. Of course, in order for people to find the personal time they need for this reflection and planning in their lives, they have to be able to take a break from their service.

This is where you can help. Perhaps you know someone who cares for an elderly parent or a disabled person, or a parent who has several small children running around the house, or even a frazzled church volunteer. This week, think about what you can do to help that person. Could you take their laundry and do it for a few weeks to give them a break? Could you come in and vacuum and dust their house? Could you deliver one meal a week for a few weeks? Could you take over some of their responsibilities at church? These are simple ideas that are truly helpful.

So today, have compassion on the compassionate. They will truly appreciate it, and you will be a part of enabling them to continue on in their roles as compassionate providers.

Dear Father of compassion, teach me Your ways. Open my eyes so I can see those around me who are hurting and tired. Help me to be willing to freely give my time to others. So little from me can mean so much to them. Amen.

REFLECTION AND APPLICATION

Dear Lord, I know that every day You demonstrate compassion to me in ways I don't always see or even understand. Thank You for always watching over me and for always being there when I am in need of Your help. Amen.

In the New Testament, the primary word used for "compassion" incorporates the idea of being moved in an emotional way when confronted with affliction. The stress on this particular word is on the action that flows out of a person's being when he or she is touched by another's suffering. Biblical compassion always leads to action.

In the parable of the Good Samaritan in Luke 10:30-36, when the Samaritan came across the wounded man, something stirred within his heart to cause him to want to help. This compassion compelled him to act on the man's behalf. And he didn't just help the man up and brush him off—he also took him on his own donkey to an inn and paid the innkeeper to take care of him.

Think about a time in your life when you were in need. How did God show you compassion in this situation?

_____

_____

_____

_____

_____

_____

Who were the people He brought into your life to provide you comfort and care?

_____

_____

_____

_____

_____

How has God demonstrated His continuing compassion to you through the members of your First Place 4 Health group?

_____

_____

_____

_____

_____

_____

How has what you learned during your time of need better enabled you to reach out with compassion to others?

_____

_____

_____

_____

_____

_____

_____

Remember that in the parable of the Good Samaritan at least two men—a priest and a Levite—passed the injured man without stopping to help. These men were both "in the ministry" and highly educated, and one would think that they would have been the likeliest candidates to stop and help the man. But God used a Samaritan—a race looked down upon by most Jews—to demonstrate His compassion.

God's compassion offers help to all those who are in need. As you conclude this week's study, say a prayer of thanks to God for His acts of compassion in your life. Ask Him to help you be more like the Samaritan in the story—always ready and willing to help regardless of who is in need or what inconvenience it might bring to yourself.

Dear Father, I want my first instinct to be one of compassion for those in need. Teach me to be more alert to the needs of those around me. Amen.

Group Prayer Requests

4 first place
health

Today's Date: _____

Name	Request

Results

_____

_____

_____

_____

_____

growing in
gentleness

SCRIPTURE MEMORY VERSE
*Take my yoke upon you and learn from me, for I am gentle
and humble in heart, and you will find rest for your souls.*
MATTHEW 11:29

In August 1996, a three-year-old boy was visiting the Brookfield Zoo in Chicago with his mother. When they reached the gorilla enclosure, the little boy, fascinated by what he saw, left his mother's side to get a closer look. He climbed the fence enclosing the area and then lost his balance. He fell into the enclosure, 18 feet below, and was knocked unconscious.

Seven curious western lowland gorillas—animals that can stand up to 6 feet tall and weigh 450 pounds—surrounded the boy. Rescuers were immediately summoned to help the boy, but before they could arrive, one of the gorillas named Binti Jua ("Daughter of the Sunshine" in Swahili), carrying her own 17-month-old baby on her back, stooped down and picked up the limp little body. What would the gorilla do?

As the onlookers watched, Binti Jua began to cradle the young boy in her arms. Then she gently carried him over to the door of the enclosure where zoo personnel could assist him. The boy spent four days in the hospital and recovered completely from the ordeal. Binti Jua was declared a hero for this incredible act of gentleness and animal altruism.

This is a perfect picture of power under the control of gentleness— something that our world needs more of today. As a culture, we need to practice gentleness in our daily lives. As believers, we especially need to pursue gentleness in all of our relationships.

Day
1

THE MEANING OF GENTLENESS

Dear God, help me to understand the true meaning of gentleness. Help me to not be overbearing and hurtful. Teach me Your way. Amen.

In the Bible, Moses provides an interesting study of this idea of power under control. Through a series of circumstances, Moses, a Hebrew, was raised in an Egyptian court. When he later saw the injustice of an Egyptian beating one of his own people, he reacted in a powerful and ungentle manner—he killed the Egyptian. Fearing he would be found out, Moses fled to the desert.

Did Moses learn a better way to handle conflict during his years spent in the desert? It would appear so. Later on, while he was leading the Israelites to the Promised Land, we read a story of how he handled a conflict with his brother and sister in a much different manner.

Read Numbers 12:1-15. What two reasons does this passage give for why Miriam and Aaron began to talk against Moses (see vv. 1-2)?

_____

_____

_____

_____

_____

Notice the parenthetical remark about Moses in verse 3. What does this imply about Moses' character at this point?

_____

_____

_____

_____

Even in the face of a personal attack, it appears that Moses remained gentle and humble in his dealings with his family and let the Lord deal with the situation. What did God say about Miriam's and Aaron's complaints (see vv. 6-8)?

_____

_____

_____

_____

When the cloud lifted from above the tent, Miriam was afflicted with a leprosy. How did Moses react to this judgment from God? How does that reaction display his gentleness (see vv. 11-13)?

_____

_____

_____

_____

As a result, what did God do (see vv. 14-15)?

_____

_____

_____

A gentle spirit can change other people's situations! In what ways are you practicing gentleness in your life?

_____

_____

_____

_____

As you conclude today's study, remember Moses' example of gentleness. Notice also that he was more concerned about preserving God's honor than his own ego—another important aspect of gentleness.

Dear God, there is strength in gentleness. I want to become a gentle person who is strong in faith and beliefs. Show me how to be that person. Amen.

JESUS, THE EPITOME OF GENTLENESS

God, I know that Your Son, Jesus, was a gentle man, but He was not weak.
Thank You for the example of Christ that You have provided to us. Amen.

Jesus had the power to do anything that He wanted on this earth. In Matthew 26:53, He said, "Do you think I cannot call on my Father, and he will at once put at my disposal more than twelve legions of angels?" Jesus was powerful, yet He chose to be gentle. In today's study, we will look at one time He explained this type of gentleness to His disciples.

Read Matthew 18:1-4. What was the disciples' question? How did Jesus demonstrate the problem with the disciples' thinking behind this question (see vv. 1-3)?

_____

_____

_____

_____

What do you think it means when Jesus said that we must "become like little children" to enter the kingdom of heaven (see v. 3)?

_____

_____

_____

_____

Immediately after completing this teaching on the kingdom of heaven, Jesus begins to tell stories that illustrate gentleness or the lack of it. Read Matthew 18:10-14. What was the main point of Jesus' story?

_____

_____

_____

_____

What characteristics did the shepherd display in this story? Explain your answer.

_____

_____

_____

_____

Read Matthew 18:23-35. Who came to the king, and what was his problem (see vv. 24-25)?

_____

_____

_____

What act of compassion did the king do for this poor fellow (see v. 27)?

_____

_____

_____

Unfortunately, the forgiven man went straight out and demanded payment of a debt owed him by another man. He was not gentle in his demands; instead, he choked the man and had him thrown in jail. The king got wind of what this man had done. What did he say and do to the first man (see v. 31-34)?

_____

_____

_____

It appears that even when we have been wronged, gentleness is still in order. We simply cannot afford the luxury of holding bitterness against another person. It is too costly to us personally to carry that burden around within us. As you conclude today's study, ask yourself if there is anything going on in your life right now that makes you feel a little (or a lot) bruised. If so, turn to the Savior to comfort you and heal your wounds. If you are comfortable doing so, consider writing down the things that have wounded you in your prayer journal.

Dear Jesus, sometimes I can be difficult and not very gentle. Help me to keep the power I have under control so others can be blessed. Amen.

Day 3 — THE GENTLENESS OF THE HOLY SPIRIT

Dear God, thank You for the Holy Spirit, who comforts us, convicts us of sin, leads us and guides us. Amen.

When the Holy Spirit came upon Jesus at His baptism, He came down as a dove—one of the most harmless and gentle creatures on the planet. The Holy Spirit will never force us to accept Jesus. Instead, He convinces us of our sin and leads us to Jesus in a gentle manner. Today, we will examine this gentle nature of the Holy Spirit.

Read John 14:16-18. What did Jesus say He would give His disciples? What would be the duration of this gift (see v. 16)?

_____

_____

_____

_____

How would the disciples know when they received this gift? What did Jesus mean when He said "the world cannot accept him, because it neither sees him nor knows him" (v. 17)?

_____

_____

_____

_____

How does Jesus' statement in verse 18 and the provision He was making for His disciples demonstrate gentleness?

_____

_____

_____

_____

Jesus refers to this gift again in John 14:26. What two things does He say this gift will provide to the believers?

_____

_____

_____

Turn to John 16:8-15. In the following table, write down the three functions of the Comforter listed in each of the verses.

Scripture	Function of the Comforter
John 16:8	
John 16:13	
John 16:14	

The Holy Spirit is often misunderstood, and it is easy to overlook the importance of His role in our lives and in the world today. It is the Holy Spirit who is at work here on earth today, and we need His help, His comfort and His teaching.

Father God, I ask that You fill me with Yourself so that others will see Jesus living in me. Please glorify Yourself in me. Amen.

LEARNING TO BE GENTLE

Lord, You are all powerful and just. I know, also, that You are gentle with those who need gentleness. Help me learn how to be gentle but strong. Amen.

We've said it before, but it bears repeating: Gentleness does not mean weakness. Gentleness is the strength of a mother caring for her child. It is the strength of a teacher who cares so much for her students that she will not allow a child to slide by with half-hearted work. It is the strength of a father who corrects his child with firmness, but does it with respect, love and understanding. Gentleness is love wrapped in character. We will look at how to develop this type of gentleness in our lives today.

Read 2 Timothy 2:14-26. In this passage, Paul is giving the younger Timothy some instruction in the faith. What important guidance does he give Timothy in verse 14? How does this relate to having gentleness?

_____

_____

_____

_____

In verse 16, Paul advises Timothy to avoid "godless chatter." How can this be seen as a prelude to gentleness?

_____

_____

_____

_____

After giving Timothy some instruction on right living, he mentions two men, Hymenaeus and Philetus, in verses 17-18. In what ways do you think these two characters are gentle or not?

_____

_____

_____

_____

Second Timothy 2:22-26 is the heart of Paul's teaching in this chapter. In the following table, look at the instruction in the left-hand column and then write down in the right-hand column how that instruction relates to becoming a gentle person.

Instruction	How it relates to becoming gentle
Flee the evil desires of youth (v. 22)	
Pursue righteousness, faith, love and peace (v. 22)	
Don't engage in foolish and stupid arguments (v. 23)	
Don't quarrel but be kind to everyone and not resentful (v. 24)	
Gently instruct those who oppose you (v. 25)	

So, what are the qualities of a gentle person? Well, gentle people find a way to be constructive even when provoked. They do not envy others. They do not need to impress others with their importance. They have manners and are not touchy. They think the best of others and exhibit Christ's love and gentleness in their own hearts and lives. Given this description, what does the fruit of gentleness look like in your life?

_____

_____

_____

_____

_____

Dear Lord, when I think of the amazing work You have done in my life,
I am so grateful for the gentle way in which the Holy Spirit has brought
me to You for forgiveness and renewal. Thank You, Lord. Amen.

FINDING REST THROUGH GENTLENESS

Dear God, help me to rest in You. Let my tired, weary soul find quiet in who You are and the ways in which You deal with Your children.

Many people today are caught in a storm of conflict, bitterness, unhappiness, dissatisfaction and sorrow. They react at the slightest provocation and take anything said to them as a personal attack. But today, God invites each of us to find rest and peace in Him. We can find that rest through gentleness.

In Matthew 11:28-30, Jesus gives us a picture of the gentle life God intends for us to live. What invitation does Jesus offer us in this passage?

_____

_____

_____

_____

In verse 29, Jesus says, "Take my yoke upon you . . . for I am gentle and humble in heart." What does it mean to take on Jesus' yoke?

_____

_____

_____

_____

A "yoke" is a device shaped to fit over the neck of load-pulling animals. It serves to link animals together so that each has the benefit of the strength of the other animals to help pull. A proper fitting yoke is vital to the ease with which oxen can pull a heavy load. Given this, what is Jesus was saying with regard to finding peace through gentleness?

_____

_____

_____

_____

Turn to Matthew 12:3-13. In this passage, the Pharisees, the religious leaders of the day, had just accused Jesus of doing work on the Sabbath because they had picked some heads of grain to eat. The yoke of the Pharisees was not easy—they had added regulation to regulation until the people could hardly move without breaking a rule. How did Jesus respond to their accusations (see vv. 3-8)?

_____

_____

_____

_____

The religious leaders then followed Jesus to a synagogue, still looking for a reason to accuse Him of breaking the Law. How did Jesus respond when they asked Him if it were lawful to heal someone on the Sabbath (see vv. 11-12)?

_____

_____

_____

How rigid are your rules for life? What rules do you have for right living that make it easy for you to be gentle with other people?

_____

_____

_____

_____

In spite of the accusations of the Pharisees, Jesus healed the man, and he went away amazed at what Jesus had done. He was the recipient of the gentleness of Jesus—no matter what day of the week it was.

Lord God, help me to be open to listening to the words of others. Help me to know when I should bend and where and when I should hold the line. Amen.

APPLICATION AND REFLECTION

*Father God, thank You for the opportunities You give to me to practice
gentleness. Let me be quick to listen and slow to become angry.*

As you know, when you are trying to lose weight, it is helpful to keep a
record of what you eat at each meal. This is because it forces you to take
a good look at what you are eating and consider whether it is a good
choice or not. In the same way, keeping a record of times when you have
exhibited gentleness can encourage you to continue developing gentleness or help you focus on any problem areas in your life.

As you look back on the past week, describe a few instances in which
you responded with gentleness when you could have chosen harshness.

_____

_____

_____

_____

Now think of a few instances when you responded the opposite—when
you just reacted instead of restraining yourself.

_____

_____

_____

_____

Which list was easier to compile? If you found more items on your "harsh
list," think about how you could have responded differently in each case.
Now pray, thanking the Lord for giving you self-control and asking the
Holy Spirit to continue to help you exhibit gentleness before you act
harshly. Ask Him to teach you how to be gentle with everyone you meet.

*Dear Lord, help me to be quick to listen, slow to speak and slow to become
angry in every situation (see James 1:19). Thank You, Lord. Amen.*

APPLICATION AND REFLECTION

Father, learning to be gentle will take vigilance on my part.
Help me not to speak or react before I have taken the time
to think about what I'm doing. Thank You, Lord God.

This week, we looked at how Jesus exhibited power under control. Although He had legions or angels at His disposal and could have done anything He wanted, He chose to be merciful and gentle.

As you have looked at this week's lesson, you may have been reminded of the times when Jesus was gentle with you when you may have deserved harshness. In the same way, it is important to extend that same grace and mercy to those in your life who might not deserve it. This is difficult to do, but with patience and practice, you can grow in gentleness.

On Day Four, we looked at Paul's words in 2 Timothy 2:24-26 as they related to exhibiting gentleness. Today, personalize this passage and pray it as a request to God, asking Him to help you in the area of gentleness. You can write down your own prayer in your journal or simply say the one below:

> *Lord, because I am Your servant, I must not quarrel but be kind to everyone. I must be willing to teach at all times and not be resentful. If there are those who oppose me, I must gently instruct them and trust that You will grant them repentance and lead them to a knowledge of the truth. I don't need to worry about their actions—You can bring them to their senses and change their hearts. Please help me, Lord, to take my clue from our gentle Savior, Jesus, and to practice gentleness in a way that pleases Him. Amen.*

Remember, Jesus said, "Come to me, all you who are weary and burdened . . . for I am gentle and humble in heart, and you will find rest for your souls" (Matthew 11:28-29). Today, seek out His gentleness and find rest in Him.

Group Prayer Requests

4 first place health

Today's Date: _____

Name	Request

Results

_____
_____
_____
_____
_____
_____

growing in
self-control

SCRIPTURE MEMORY VERSE
*So I say, live by the Spirit, and you will not gratify
the desires of the sinful nature.*
GALATIANS 5:16

Anyone who has attempted to lead a balanced lifestyle ultimately realizes that good choices are made by exerting self-control. When we walk into a grocery store, self-control whispers to us that we can't head straight for the ice cream aisle to fill up our cart with our favorite flavors. It says we can't eat triple cheeseburgers at our favorite fast food restaurant every day. Self-control tells us that we can't give into the temptation to lounge on the sofa instead of exercising because the weather is bad outside or we just don't feel like doing our fitness routine.

Steve Reynolds, a pastor in Virginia, has been called "the anti-fat pastor" by the media. Steve was seriously overweight, and his health was being threatened by high blood pressure and diabetes. For a while after his diagnosis, Steve didn't realize that he might be able to do something to help his health situation if he were to lose weight and exercise. When he finally realized that he could improve his situation if he made some changes, he began to use self-control to eat what he calls "live food"—the type of food that has to be replaced when it reaches its expiration date. It's not the packaged, processed, chemical-loaded food we find on the aisles of the grocery store.

Steve also began to exercise every day. He eventually started a program in his church called "Bod4God," where participants learned how to eat and exercise and encouraged each other to lose weight. People in Steve's church have since lost hundreds and hundreds of pounds. Steve himself dropped 110 pounds, and he was able to stop taking both diabetes and blood pressure medicine.

As Christians, each of us has the Holy Spirit prompting and encouraging us to exert self-control. The Holy Spirit is an expert in growing this fruit of the Spirit in our lives. This week, we will look at how this occurs.

Day 1   FOLLOW THE RULES

Dear God, teach me to walk in Your path and do Your will at all times. Warn me when I've started down the wrong path and bring me back to walking in obedience. Amen.

In any venture, if you don't follow the rules, you risk suffering the consequences. For instance, if you are driving down the road and decide not to stop at a red light, the consequences can be quite serious. Likewise, having self-control requires knowing the rules set forth in the Bible and following them. It is God's holy Word to us, and it teaches us how to live. Today, we will examine what the Bible says about itself.

Read Psalm 119:1-8. Where can we find the statutes, precepts and decrees referred to in this passage?

_____

_____

_____

_____

Why does the psalmist say these things are important in our lives?

_____

_____

_____

_____

Read Psalm 119:9-13. In verse 9, the psalmist asks, "How can a young man keep his way pure? By living according to your word." In what ways does living according to the Word help you keep your life pure?

_____

_____

_____

_____

Of what advantage is it to us to hide God's Word in our hearts?

_____

_____

_____

Read Psalm 119:14-16. How does the psalmist describe his response to the statutes, precepts and decrees given in the Word of God?

_____

_____

_____

_____

The psalmist states he delights in God's decrees and will not neglect God's Word. This writer knew the rulebook, and he took great delight in studying it. In light of these 16 verses of Scripture, in what ways would you say that you know the rulebook and are playing by those rules? How might you improve your knowledge of God's Word?

_____

_____

_____

_____

Dear God, thank You for Your Word, the Book that gives life's instructions.
Help me to love Your Word the way that the psalmist loved it. Amen.

Day
2
THE RESULTS OF LACKING SELF-CONTROL

Dear God, Your Word has a story or teaching to guide me in every
situation in life. Help me to learn from the tragic stories as well as from
those that bring me joy. Amen.

America is facing a growing problem, and it is occurring right within our homes: childhood obesity. In one study, researchers discovered that children who exhibited low self-control at age 3 were much more likely by age 12 to suffer problems from weight than those who had higher self-control. The study also found that children with low self-control not only gained more weight than the others but also gained it faster.[1]

The lesson to be learned is obvious: Parents have to teach their kids how to have self-control. Of course, the best way to teach anything to children is to model good behavior. This means that parents must first practice self-control in their own lives in order to then be able to model it for their kids.

A lack of self-control always causes problems. Today, we will look at how a lack of self-control caused problems in one famous king's family in the Bible.

Read 2 Samuel 13:1-19. What was Amnon's "problem" (see vv. 1-2)?

_____

_____

_____

_____

A friend of Amnon's hatched a plot to help his friend. What was the plot (see vv. 3-6)?

_____

_____

_____

_____

_____

While Amnon's friend's plan may not have had evil as its intent, Amnon's lack of self-control came into play. What evil thing did this cause him to do (see vv. 10-14)?

_____

_____

_____

_____

As soon as Amnon had indulged his lack of self-control, his attitude toward Tamar changed drastically. What happened (see v. 15)?

_____

_____

_____

_____

As soon as Amnon had what he thought he wanted, he despised what he had gained through his lack of self-control. When you lose control of your life and indulge yourself, how do you feel? Is the indulgence worth the emotional price you pay afterward?

_____

_____

_____

_____

James 1:15 says, "Then, after desire has conceived, it gives birth to sin; and sin, when it is full-grown, gives birth to death." The result of having low self-control and giving in to desires is serious business. How do you plan to increase your self-control so that you can lead a healthy and more balanced life?

_____

_____

_____

_____

Dear God, thank You for the gift of self-control. Holy Spirit, please con-
tinue to grow this fruit in my life. Help me every time I face temptation to
listen for Your voice encouraging me to have self-control. Amen.

Day
3

A LIFE OF SELF-CONTROL

Dear God, I need more self-control in my life. Please teach me Your way,
for truly, self-control is Holy-Spirit control. Help me to listen for
Your voice and Your teaching. Amen.

Often, the problem with self-control is that although we know what we should do—what is the right choice—we act before we think. Something happens that triggers an emotional reaction, and off we go. Or we are impulsive and rush to make a decision before we have all the facts. Seeing self-control as something unpleasant can also set up a barrier in embracing this in our life. Yet self-control is a discipline that is needed in the Christian life. When it is used wisely, it can become one of the more important tools for self-improvement and achieving success.

One of the best measures of how well we do in this area of self-control is how well we control our speech. In his epistle, James speaks about the need for us as Christians to have control over our tongue. We will study this aspect of self-control today.

Read James 3:1-8. At the beginning of this passage, James says that we all stumble in many ways, and then he describes the perfect person. What is the perfect person able to do (see v. 2)?

_____

_____

_____

_____

_____

_____

James uses the example of horses to describe something that must be controlled. What must we do to get horses to obey us (see v. 3)?

_____

_____

_____

_____

James also uses an example of a ship to illustrate this same point. What must we do to keep a ship from floundering (see v. 4)?

_____

_____

_____

_____

The bit and the rudder are small parts, but they are important. How does James say the tongue is similar (see v. 5)?

_____

_____

_____

How is the tongue like a fire? What does James mean when he says that it "corrupts the whole person" (v. 6)?

_____

_____

_____

_____

Why is it that "no man can tame the tongue" (v. 8)? Who can tame it?

_____

_____

_____

_____

The tongue displays what it going on in the heart. If we have trouble keeping our tongue under control, we may need to look deeper into our heart and soul to see what is really going on.

> *Lord, I confess that sometimes I lack self-control. Help me find a way to let Your Spirit control my life. Please give me the key to overcoming any weakness in this area and help me react with self-control in every situation. Amen.*

Day 4 | THE BLESSING OF SELF-CONTROL

Dear God, help me to help others as I learn self-control. Let me be a blessing in a world that is hurting, because many people are constantly on the edge of losing control. May you be glorified through my life and my actions. Amen.

Whether you define character as humility, work ethic or making healthful choices, self-control—the ability to delay gratification and choose what is right even when it is difficult to do so—is always required in the mix. It is the cornerstone of all facets of a person's character.[2]

Self-control benefits ourselves and others because it grows character in us and enables us to display many qualities that are needed in the world today. Self-control grows kindness. It is at the heart of goodness and is a component of humility. It compels us to work hard at whatever task is at hand and to make healthy choices.

Today, we will look at what the apostle Paul said to the believers in the church in Corinth in regard to building character and how this was a direct result of their ability to have self-control.

Read 1 Corinthians 3:1-9. What is Paul's complaint against the Corinthians (see vv. 1-3)?

_____

_____

_____

_____

Quarreling and jealousy certainly don't speak of self-control. These are actions that speak of a lack of control and of speaking out before thinking. What seems to be the issue about which the Corinthian believers were arguing (see v. 4)?

_____

_____

_____

_____

_____

What does Paul say on this matter? What was his and Apollos's task? How was God using each of them (see vv. 5-9)?

_____

_____

_____

_____

_____

Read 1 Corinthians 3:16-18. In this passage, Paul reminds the Corinthian believers that each of them is a temple of God. What warning does he then give them (see v. 17)?

_____

_____

_____

How should self-control be exhibited in the life of someone who is a temple of God?

_____

_____

_____

_____

What does Paul say about wisdom in verse 18?

_____

_____

_____

_____

Wisdom and the ability to have self-control are closely related. When we embrace this fruit of the Spirit in our lives, we will not overreact at the slightest provocation but take the time to think through the situation and then act in a wise manner. In the process, we will avoid offending others by not flying off the handle and saying things that we later regret. Such practices will build character in us and serve to bless others.

> *Dear God, I know that when I lose control I often hurt others with what I say. Help me, for I am in need of Your strength, wisdom and guidance in how to become self-controlled. Amen.*

Day 5

THE MODEL FOR SELF-CONTROL

Dear God, Your Son, Jesus, is the perfect model for almost every character trait we need to develop. Help me to be like Him. Amen.

Jesus had many opportunities to lose control and strike back at those who criticized Him while He was on earth. Yet time and again, we see Him facing false accusations, injustices and personal injury and not losing control. Even when He was truly angry at the moneychangers in the Temple and overturned their tables, there is no indication that He ever lost control of Himself. He was displaying a righteous anger against the sin He saw in His Father's house.

This should give each of us great hope, for we know that He lives in each one of us and can help us to become more like Him. Today, we will look at another example of Jesus' self-control, which took place shortly after His arrest when He was put on trial.

Read Mark 14:53-65. What were the chief priests hoping to accomplish by bringing Jesus to trial before them? What measures did they take to accomplish this (see vv. 55-56)?

_____

_____

_____

_____

_____

What was the witnesses' main complaint against him? What was the problem with their testimony? What does this fact indicate to you (see vv. 57-59)?

_____

_____

_____

_____

What do you think you might have said or done if you had been standing there listening to a barrage of lies about your purpose?

_____

_____

_____

_____

How did Jesus react to these accusations (see v. 61)? What does this demonstrate about His character?

_____

_____

_____

_____

Read Mark 15:1-5. After the trial before the Sanhedrin, Jesus was taken to Pilate for a repeat performance of the accusations and lies. What was Jesus' response? What did Pilate think about Jesus' response (see vv. 4-5)?

_____

_____

_____

_____

How did this conversation show self-control on the part of Jesus?

_____

_____

_____

_____

The bloodthirsty crowd certainly did not display self-control. They raged against Jesus, shouting for Him to be crucified. The Roman soldiers spat at Him, blindfolded Him, struck Him with their fists and mocked Him. If anyone had a right to strike back against the treatment He received, it would have been Jesus. Yet He exercised self-control and went through the ordeal of the cross so that we could be free from the power of sin and death.

> *Jesus, thank You for what You did for me. Thank You for maintaining self-control even in this situation. I love You for dying on the cross for me. Amen.*

Day 6

APPLICATION AND REFLECTION

Dear Lord, I want to put into practice what I've learned about self-control. Guide me toward self-discipline and self-control. Amen.

Today, think about your own situation. What scenarios cause you to "blow your top" and lose control? Who is it that bugs you until you almost can't stand it? What situation or circumstance irritates you every time it happens? When does temptation get the best of you? Mentally walk yourself through that experience and think about how you typically react. Now, write down a plan for how you will overcome that situation. Describe what you will do the next time you are confronted with the troublesome person or circumstance.

_____

_____

_____

_____

Finally, say a prayer, asking the Lord to help you to be victorious in your life and overcome the attacks of the enemy when he tempts you to lose control.

Dear Lord, I need more of Your power in my life. Please take complete control of my situation—I give it up completely to You and rest in Your comfort and grace. Amen.

APPLICATION AND REFLECTION

Day 7

Dear God, thank You for the fruit of the Spirit that You have planted in my life. Help me to do what I must to have a fruitful harvest. Lead me day by day closer to You. Thank You, Lord. Amen.

This week we have focused on learning self-control, but the truth is that as believers, we must be under the leading, teaching and inspiration of the Holy Spirit in all areas of our spiritual growth. We must seek out this growth and continually ask God to develop each fruit of the Spirit in our lives. We must also look to the example of Jesus as our model for how to live out each of these fruits.

Something you might do to remind yourself that God is slowly growing His fruit in you is to get a pot and plant something in it and watch it grow. See how long it takes for the fruit of the plant to develop and ripen. Even if what you plant is a flower, there is a process whereby the flower turns into a seed-bearing fruit. It all takes time, but little by little, the fruit appears and matures.

Today, take one final look at all the fruit of the Spirit and evaluate the progress you have made these past 11 weeks toward growth in each.

Spiritual fruit	My progress
Love	
Joy	
Peace	
Patience	
Kindness	
Goodness	
Faithfulness	
Compassion	
Gentleness	
Self-control	

growing in self-control | 165

After you have completed your reflection, end your quiet time by thanking the Lord for revealing Himself in new and exciting ways as you have studied His Word and lived in His mercy and grace.

Dear God, what a great idea You had when You decided to grow these fruit of the Spirit in our lives. Let me make every day for the rest of my life a time when I am nurturing one or more of these fruit. Thank You, Lord! Amen.

Notes
1. Alice Park, "Kids Who Lack Self-Control More Prone to Obesity Later," Time, April 7, 2009. http://www.time.com/time/health/article/0,8599,1889942,00.html.
2. Dr. Joseph J. Horton, Dr. Kevin S. Seybold and Dr. Gary L. Welton, "Social Organizations as a Path to Self-Control: Does Religious Participation Promote Character Development?" December 23, 2008, Grove City College. http://www.visandvals.org/Social_Organizations_as_a_Path_to_Self_control.php.

Group Prayer Requests

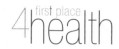

Today's Date: _____

Name	Request

Results

_____

_____

_____

_____

_____

_____

time to
celebrate!

To help shape your brief victory celebration testimony, work through the following questions in your prayer journal:

Day One: List some of the benefits you have gained by allowing the Lord to transform your life through this 12-week First Place 4 Health session. Be sure to list benefits you have received in the physical, mental, emotional and spiritual realms of your being.

Day Two: In what ways have you most significantly changed *mentally*? Have you seen a shift in the ways you think about yourself, food, your relationships or God? How has Scripture memory been a part of these shifts?

Day Three: In what ways have you most significantly changed *emotionally*? Have you begun to identify how your feelings influence your relationship to food and exercise? What are you doing to stay aware of your emotions, both positive and negative?

Day Four: In what ways have you most significantly changed *spiritually*? How has your relationship with God deepened? How has drawing closer to Him made a difference in the other three areas of your life?

Day Five: In what ways have you most significantly changed *physically*? Have you met or exceeded your weight/measurement goals? How has your health improved in the past 12 weeks?

Day Six: Was there one person in your First Place 4 Health group who was particularly encouraging to you? How did their kindness make a difference in your First Place 4 Health journey?

Day Seven: Summarize the previous six questions into a one-page testimony, or "faith story," to share at your group's victory celebration.

May our gracious Lord bless and keep you as you continue to keep Him first in all things!

Growing in the Fruit of the Spirit
leader discussion guide

For in-depth information, guidance and helpful tips about leading a successful First Place 4 Health group, study the *First Place 4 Health Leader's Guide*. In it, you will find valuable answers to most of your questions, as well as personal insights from many First Place 4 Health group leaders.

For the group meetings in this session, be sure to read and consider each week's discussion topics several days before the meeting—some questions and activities require supplies and/or planning to complete. Also, if you are leading a large group, plan to break into smaller groups for discussion and then come together as a large group to share your answers and responses. Make sure to appoint a capable leader for each small group so that discussions stay focused and on track (and be sure each group records their answers!).

week one: welcome to *Growing in the Fruit of the Spirit*
During this first week, welcome the members to your group, provide a brief overview of the First Place 4 Health program, explain what is expected of the participants at each of the weekly meetings, and collect the Member Surveys. (See the *First Place 4 Health Leader's Guide* for a detailed outline of how to conduct the first week's meeting.)

week two: growing in love
Ask participants to discuss the arguments that John makes in 1 John 4:7-21 for why we should love one another. Talk about what John says about those who do not show love.

Discuss the concept of the sin offering from the Day Two study. Ask the members in what way Jesus served as the "atoning sacrifice" for our sins and how Jesus' death on the cross was the fulfillment of God's love for humankind.

Have someone in the group read 1 John 3:16. Ask the members if laying down their lives would be something they could honestly say they would be willing to do for another. Why or why not?

Discuss the differences between *phileo* and *agape* love. Talk about how *agape* love is the self-sacrificing love that Jesus demonstrated and how it enables us to love our enemies and those who are difficult in our lives.

Ask the members to recount the main point that Jesus was trying to make to Peter when He asked Peter three times if he truly loved Him. What type of love was Jesus talking about when He asked this question? What type of response was Peter giving?

Discuss what Jesus' command after each question to "feed my lambs" indicates about how each of us should demonstrate love.

During the Day Five study, the members read Paul's words in 1 Corinthians 13:13: "And now these three remain: faith, hope and love. But the greatest of these is love." Discuss why Paul believed love to be the greatest gift of God.

Close with a time of prayer. Encourage members to pray that God will reveal His love in their lives and that He will help them to share His love with others.

week three: growing in hope

This week, the members read the story of Job. Have the group discuss what misfortunes he experienced and what his response was to God. Talk about the fact that even though Job went through immense suffering, he was able to maintain his hope in God.

On Day One, the participants were asked to look up Psalms 25:3; 33:18; 33:20 and 147:11 and write down the promise they found in each one as it relates to hope. Have different people in the group read each verse, and then have the members discuss what they found.

On Day Two, the members read about how Abraham, "against all hope," believed in God's promise that he would have a son. Discuss why God might have had Abraham wait so long before the promise was fulfilled.

Discuss what God did for Abraham during this period of waiting to encourage him to keep hoping. Ask the members if they are hoping and waiting for something to come to pass in their lives. If so, how has God encouraged them to keep hoping and trusting in Him during this time?

On Day Three, the members studied how they can obtain hope in their own lives. Discuss what Paul says in Romans about what their responsibility is to carry out that hope. What does God say that He will do for us and in us in these verses?

Discuss how each of us as Christians can be sure that no matter what happens here on earth, we have the hope of eternal life. How should knowing this fact change the way each of us deals with the problems and trials that we go through each day?

Conclude with a time of prayer. Encourage members to thank God for this gift of hope and to pray that He will help them to never lose sight of it when difficult times come.

week four: growing in faith

Ask the members what was unique about the centurion's response in Matthew 8:5-13 when Jesus said He would come to heal His servant. How did that response demonstrate faith? How did Jesus react when He heard the centurion's statement?

On Day Two, the members read about the faith of the woman who "touched" Jesus in Luke 8:40-48. Discuss how her action of touching Jesus required a great deal of faith on her part.

Have the group share one person from the "Hall of Faith" in Hebrews 11 that especially interested them. In what ways did the writer of Hebrews commend that individual for their faith?

Discuss some of the benefits each of us receives here on earth from having faith in God. Ask one or two members to share a story of how faith in God has helped them get through a difficult situation or given them strength when they needed it the most.

Discuss what Jesus meant by the statement, "It is easier for a camel to go through the eye of a needle than for a rich man to enter the kingdom of God" (Matthew 19:24).

What did Jesus reveal to Peter about the disciples' (and our) coming rewards in heaven?

Conclude with a time of prayer, thanking God for the gift of faith and asking Him to help the members to be confident in sharing that faith with others.

week five: growing in goodness

Discuss some of the good things that David says the Lord does for us in Psalm 23:1-3. In what ways does the "rod" and the "staff" of God bring comfort to us?

Have the group share some of the qualities of goodness that Jesus discussed in Luke 6:27-35. Why would Jesus' statement in verse 27, "Love your enemies, do good to those who hate you," have been controversial?

In Luke 6:29, when Jesus says to "turn to him the other [cheek] also," what He is really talking about is a punch in the jaw. Discuss the type of heart attitude that Jesus is stating we must adopt in this verse.

Discuss what Jesus meant when He said that we must be like "salt" and "light" to others. How are we to affect our environment?

Have someone in the group read Galatians 5:24-26. Discuss what steps we need to take based on Paul's words in this passage about how we can allow God's goodness to be in us. What things do we have to clear from our lives? What things must we embrace to live a life of goodness?

Have a few members in the group give some of the examples they found in the Day Five study about the types of good works that Jesus did while on earth. Ask if there was any one particular deed that stood out for them and, if so, why this was the case.

Conclude with a time of prayer, asking God to help the members continue to grow in goodness and reflect the light of God to the people in their lives.

week six: growing in joy

Discuss some of the ways that David describes the Lord in Psalm 71. How does David express his joy in the Lord?

When the angels came to announce the birth of Christ to the shepherds, they said, "I bring you good news of great joy" (Luke 2:10). Ask the group why they think the angels described the birth of Christ as "good news of great joy." What did Christ represent to the world?

Discuss some of the ways that David states in Psalm 51:1-19 about what we should be requesting from God to receive new joy. What were some of his specific requests in this passage?

If they are comfortable in doing so, have a few members in the group share a situation when they felt they needed God to restore the joy of their salvation. What caused the loss of joy?

On Day Three, the members read about a problem going on in the church at Philippi (see Philippians 4:2-7). Discuss what this problem was and what Paul's advice was to the church on how to resolve it.

Have the group comment on what was unique about Paul's situation when he wrote this letter to the Philippians. Discuss how despite being in chains, he was able to rejoice in his immediate situation. What did Paul find to rejoice about in this situation?

Ask the members to honestly think about how they would most likely react if they were in a similar situation. (If time allows, you could have one or two people discuss a hardship in their lives that they are experiencing right now and how God could use that situation to bring joy in their lives.) How can we choose to deliberately rejoice in any situation?

Conclude with a time of prayer, praising God for the joy He has provided to each of us and for the incredible sacrifice of His Son that allows us to experience that joy.

week seven: growing in peace

On Day One, the group members looked up several passages about peace (Psalm 29:11; Isaiah 26:3; John 16:33; Romans 15:13). Have those in the group read these verses aloud, and then discuss some of the answers they wrote down on where to find peace.

Ask the group to talk about any of the "peace wreckers" they looked at during the Week Two study that particularly resonated with them. Are they currently experiencing any of these peace wreckers in their lives?

Discuss some of the arguments Paul had with Peter (see Galatians 2:11) and Barnabas (see Acts 15:37-38). What was the result of these disagreements? Was it okay for these early leaders in the Church to disagree with each other? Why or why not?

Have members read one passage of Scripture from the Day Three study that discusses peace (Leviticus 19:28; Galatians 5:13; Colossians 3:14; James 1:19; 1 Peter 2:17; 1 Peter 3:8; 1 Peter 4:8) and briefly comment on how that passage provides instruction for restoring peace.

Paul, even though he had persecuted Christians, was able to accept the complete forgiveness of Christ and radically turn about to a new life. Discuss how Paul was able to forgive himself for the things he had done and how he now viewed his status in Christ (see Ephesians 1:4-5,18-19).

Ask those in the group if there is anything from their past they are continuing to drag around with them. Is there anything they have confessed but are still feeling guilty about? Based on what they studied this week, is this something that God wants them to do? Why or why not?

Discuss some of the reasons Scripture gives for why we are to pray for peace (see Jeremiah 29:7; Ephesians 2:14-22; Colossians 3:15). What does the Bible tell us to do when we pray for peace? What is Christ trying to build here on earth?

Conclude with a time of prayer, asking God to continue to help the members seek peace with those in their lives and to restore any relationship that might have been broken over disagreements they might have had with others.

week eight: growing in patience

On Day One, the group members revisited the story of Abraham and Sarah to examine some of the problems they had with being patient as they waited for God's promise of a son to arrive. Discuss from the reading in Genesis 16:1-4 what Sarah did that flew in the face of God's promise. How was this an act of impatience?

Discuss the result of Sarah's impatience as it relates to her relationship with Hagar. What were the consequences of Abraham and Sarah's impatience? What can that teach us about waiting on God's timing?

On Day Two, the members looked at some passages of Scripture relating to patience. Have different members read Proverbs 19:11; Ecclesiastes 7:8 and Colossians 1:9-12 and discuss what they discovered about how each of us can grow in this fruit of the Spirit.

Have someone in the group read James 1:2-4. Discuss why James states we should consider trials of many kinds "pure joy." What is the purpose of developing perseverance according to this passage?

Have someone in the group read Romans 5:3-4. Ask the group how Paul's words affirm this idea that we must go through some periods of suffering to learn patience.

Discuss some of the ways from the Day Four study in which Noah had to persevere in order to follow the instructions he had been given from God. In what ways might he have felt singled out and separated from others? Would he have felt lonely? What does this tell us about some of the times when we will have to persevere to follow God?

Discuss how Jacob struggled with patience and how he often took matters into his own hands. What problems did this often cause for him? What was it that Jacob wanted that ultimately led to him being willing to learn patience (see Genesis 29:16-27)? How did this situation help him learn how to persevere?

Close with a time of prayer. Encourage members to pray that God will continue to help them develop patience and perseverance in their lives.

week nine: growing in compassion

Ask the members to discuss what Paul says about the compassion of God the Father in 2 Corinthians 1:3-7. For what reason does God comfort us in our troubles? How is compassion closely connected to the concept of *agape* love that the members studied during Week Two?

Discuss what Jesus meant when He said, "Blessed are the meek" (Matthew 5:5). Who were the "meek" in Jesus' time? In what ways did Christ specifically target these groups during His ministry on earth?

Ask a few people in the group to read the passages of Scripture from the Day Three study that describe some of Christ's acts of compassion (Matthew 9:35-36, 20:29-34; Mark 1:40-42; John 11:17-36; 12:3-7). Have them explain how Jesus' action demonstrated God's compassion.

Discuss with the group the ways in which Jesus showed compassion to them specifically as individuals. In what ways do they need His compassion in their lives right now?

On Day Four, the members read how we are often like sheep who get lost and go astray. Discuss in what ways we are in need of a compassionate shepherd in our lives. Why does Jesus refer to Himself as "the good shepherd" who "lays down his life for the sheep" (John 10:11)?

Ask the members to list some of the practical ways they have reached out to people with compassion in the past. How did doing this act make them feel? In what way can they envision what they did to be an act of God's love to this world?

Ask if any members of the group know someone who has suffered from "compassion fatigue." If so, what are some ways they would be willing to help these individuals? What can the group do as a whole to identify those people in the church who are in danger of compassion burnout?

Close with a time of prayer, asking God to continue to help members model the actions of Jesus while He was on earth and extend the gift of compassion to others. Say a prayer thanking God for the compassion that He extends to each of us every day.

week ten: growing in gentleness

Discuss the ways in which Moses was "ungentle" toward the Egyptian who was beating one of the Hebrews and the result of his action. How did Moses handle the situation differently in Numbers 12:1-15 when his brother and sister began to complain against him? What does that tell us about how a gentle spirit can change another person's actions?

Discuss some of the characteristics of Jesus' gentleness. Was Jesus weak or powerful? In what ways did He demonstrate power under the control of mercy?

Briefly discuss the parable of the unmerciful servant in Matthew 18:23-35. Based on this parable, when we have been wronged, how does God expect us to act toward others? Why does He expect this?

Ask the participants to discuss the significance of the Holy Spirit coming down in the form of a dove when Jesus was baptized. What did this symbolically represent? What does this tell us about His nature?

Ask the group members to discuss some of the functions of the "Comforter" that they found in John 16:8,13-14. Why is the function of the Holy Spirit so often misunderstood?

Discuss how Paul's words to Timothy in 2 Timothy 2:22-26 relate to us becoming more gentle people. How can we begin to implement Paul's instruction into our lives? What things are we to embrace to grow in gentleness? What things are we to avoid?

As the participants read in the Day Five study, a "yoke" serves to link animals together so that each has the benefit of the strength of the other animals in the yoke to help pull. Given this explanation, discuss what Jesus was saying in Matthew 11:29 when He said, "Take my yoke upon you . . . for I am gentle and humble in heart." What was Jesus saying with regard to finding peace through gentleness?

Close with a time of prayer, asking God to continue to help members exhibit power under the control of gentleness. Say a prayer of thanksgiving to God that He is always gentle and patient with us.

week eleven: growing in self-control

Ask the participants to discuss some of the consequences they have personally seen in their lives as it pertains to a lack of self-control. How do they plan to increase their self-control so that they can lead a healthy and more balanced life? What is their role in this? What is God's role in this?

Have the group look at some of the examples of the tongue from the Day Three study that James lists in James 3:1-8. What do the examples of the horse and the ship tell us about the power of our words? What does the bit and the rudder tell us about the importance of the tongue? In what ways is the tongue like a fire?

Discuss what Paul's primary complaint was against the Corinthian believers in 1 Corinthians 3:1-9. What things were they doing that did not demonstrate good self-control? How should the discipline of self-control be exhibited in the life of someone who is a "temple of God"?

Discuss some of the ways Jesus demonstrated self-control in Mark 14:53-65. What was happening to Him in this situation? What does the witnesses' testimony tells us about the accuracy and fairness of what they were saying? How did Jesus react in the face of these false accusations?

Ask the group to discuss any situations they have experienced recently in which they felt they were not being fairly treated. How did it make them feel? How did they react? If they did show self-control, ask them to share how they were able to do this. If not, ask them to share their ideas for how they wished they had handled the situation differently.

On Day Six, the members were asked to list specific scenarios that cause them to "blow their top" and lose control. Ask a few participants who are willing to read their responses. What plan did they come up with to help them exhibit better self-control in the future? How could this same plan be used as it relates to controlling what they eat?

Close with a time of prayer, thanking God that He has given us the power to resist temptation and exhibit self-control in our lives. Encourage the members to pray that God will enable them to grow even more in self-control so that they can truly lead balanced and healthy lives.

week twelve: time to celebrate!

Even though most of your meeting this week will be a victory celebration, take some time at the beginning of the meeting to talk about how much God loves each person in the group and how each of us is called to love our brothers and sisters in Christ. (See "Planning a Victory Celebration" in the *First Place 4 Health Leader's Guide* for ideas about throwing a successful celebration for your group.)

For the rest of the study time, allow each member to tell his or her *Growing in the Fruit of the Spirit* story. Give members an equal opportunity to share the goals they set for themselves at the beginning of the session and talk about the challenges and good things God has done for them throughout the process. Don't allow the more talkative group members to monopolize all the time—the quiet members also need an opportunity to share their stories and successes! Note that even those who have not met their goals have still been part of the journey, so be sure to allow them to share and talk about why they did not succeed.

Making a commitment to continue in First Place 4 Health is an important part of victory. Be sure to talk about your group's future plans, and make each person feel welcome to continue the journey with you.

First Place 4 Health menu plans

Each menu plan is based on approximately 1,400 to 1,500 calories per day. All recipe and menu exchanges were determined using the Master-Cook software, a program that accesses a database containing more than 6,000 food items prepared using the United States Department of Agriculture (USDA) publications and information from food manufacturers. As with any nutritional program, MasterCook calculates the nutritional values of the recipes based on ingredients. Nutrition may vary due to how the food is prepared, where the food comes from, soil content, season, ripeness, processing and method of preparation. For these reasons, please use the recipes and menu plans as approximate guides. Consult a physician and/or a registered dietitian before starting a weight-loss program.

For those who need more calories, add the following to the 1,400-calorie plan:

- 1,800 calories: 2 ounce equivalent of meat, 3 ounce equivalent of bread, $^1/_2$ cup vegetable serving, 1 tsp. fat

- 2,000 calories: 2 ounce equivalent of meat, 4 ounce equivalent of bread, $^1/_2$ cup vegetable serving, 3 tsp. fat

- 2,200 calories: 2 ounce equivalent of meat, 5 ounce equivalent of bread, $^1/_2$ cup vegetable serving, $^1/_2$ cup fruit serving, 5 tsp. fat

- 2,400 calories: 2 ounce equivalent of meat, 6 ounce equivalent of bread, 1 cup vegetable serving, $^1/_2$ cup fruit serving, 6 tsp. fat

First Week Grocery List

Produce
- [ ] asparagus
- [ ] bananas
- [ ] bell pepper
- [ ] blackberries
- [ ] blueberries
- [ ] carrots
- [ ] celery
- [ ] cucumbers
- [ ] garlic cloves
- [ ] grapefruit
- [ ] green chilies
- [ ] green peppers
- [ ] honeydew melon
- [ ] iceberg lettuce
- [ ] jalapenos
- [ ] mangos
- [ ] mushrooms
- [ ] onions
- [ ] oranges
- [ ] potatoes
- [ ] Spanish onion
- [ ] spinach
- [ ] spring mix salad
- [ ] strawberries
- [ ] sweet potatoes
- [ ] tarragon, fresh
- [ ] tomatoes
- [ ] zucchini

Baking Products
- [ ] all-fruit spread (strawberry)
- [ ] balsamic vinegar
- [ ] basil
- [ ] basil, dry leaf
- [ ] bay leaves
- [ ] black pepper, freshly ground
- [ ] brown mustard, spicy
- [ ] bouillon cubes, chicken, no-added salt
- [ ] bouillon, instant chicken or beef, low-sodium
- [ ] buttermilk baking mix, reduced-fat
- [ ] canola oil
- [ ] chili powder
- [ ] cinnamon
- [ ] cocktail sauce
- [ ] cumin
- [ ] dressing, light
- [ ] dry mustard
- [ ] garlic powder
- [ ] ketchup
- [ ] molasses
- [ ] mustard
- [ ] mustard, dry
- [ ] nonstick cooking spray
- [ ] olive oil
- [ ] oregano
- [ ] oregano, dry leaf
- [ ] paprika
- [ ] pepper
- [ ] poppy seeds
- [ ] pretzels
- [ ] raisins
- [ ] red wine vinegar
- [ ] rice
- [ ] rice mix, long grain and wild (1 pkg.)
- [ ] rosemary, fresh
- [ ] salsa
- [ ] salt
- [ ] salt, seasoned
- [ ] stuffing mix, herb-seasoned
- [ ] sugar
- [ ] syrup, sugar-free
- [ ] vanilla
- [ ] vegetable oil
- [ ] Worcestershire sauce

Breads and Cereals

- [ ] bagels
- [ ] bread, cinnamon-raisin
- [ ] bread, pumpernickel
- [ ] bread, whole-wheat
- [ ] cornbread
- [ ] corn tortillas
- [ ] crackers
- [ ] flour tortillas, lowfat (10-in.)
- [ ] French bread
- [ ] hamburger buns
- [ ] melba toast
- [ ] spaghetti
- [ ] 8 oz. tortellini, dry with Parmesan cheese (1 pkg.)

Canned Foods

- [ ] chicken broth, fat-free, reduced sodium
- [ ] cream of celery soup, reduced fat (1 can)
- [ ] cream of chicken soup, reduced fat (2 cans)
- [ ] mushrooms (1 can)
- [ ] 15½ oz. red kidney beans, low-sodium (1 can)
- [ ] 10 oz. rotel tomatoes (1 can)
- [ ] 16 oz. stewed tomatoes, low-sodium (1 can)
- [ ] 12½ oz. tomatoes, low sodium (1 can)
- [ ] tropical mixed fruit (1 can)
- [ ] 46 oz. vegetable juice (1 can)
- [ ] water chestnuts (1 can)

Dairy Products

- [ ] American cheese, light
- [ ] Asiago cheese
- [ ] cheddar cheese, reduced-fat
- [ ] Colby cheese
- [ ] Cool Whip Lite®
- [ ] cream cheese, fat-free
- [ ] eggs
- [ ] egg substitute
- [ ] feta cheese
- [ ] margarine, reduced-calorie
- [ ] mayonnaise, light
- [ ] milk, fat-free
- [ ] orange juice
- [ ] Parmesan cheese
- [ ] sour cream, nonfat
- [ ] Swiss cheese
- [ ] Velveeta® processed cheese, light
- [ ] yogurt, light
- [ ] yogurt, plain nonfat

Frozen Foods

- [ ] 10 oz. green beans, French cut (1 pkg.)
- [ ] pancakes, lowfat
- [ ] peas
- [ ] 10 oz. spinach (1 pkg.)
- [ ] waffles, lowfat

Meat and Poultry

- [ ] Canadian bacon
- [ ] chicken (with bones and skin)
- [ ] chicken breasts, boneless, skinless
- [ ] ground beef, 90-percent lean
- [ ] 2 oz. ground turkey
- [ ] 2 oz. ham, lean
- [ ] 1¼ lbs. round- or top-sirloin steaks, boneless
- [ ] 1½ oz. turkey breasts
- [ ] seafood entrée
- [ ] 2½ oz. shrimp, peeled and deveined

First Week Meals and Recipes

DAY 1

Breakfast

Breakfast Pie

nonstick cooking spray
1/2 cup chopped onion
1/2 cup chopped zucchini
2 oz. cooked mushrooms
2 oz. lean ham
1/2 cup shredded reduced-fat
 cheddar cheese

1 cup fat-free milk
2 tbsp. nonfat sour cream
2 eggs or 3 egg whites
3/4 cup reduced-fat buttermilk
 baking mix
a pinch of pepper

Preheat oven to 350° F. Spray a 9-inch pie plate with cooking spray. Spray a skillet with cooking spray; add onion, zucchini, mushrooms and ham. Cook about 2 minutes until onions are translucent. Spread onion mixture over bottom of pie plate. Sprinkle cheese on top. In a bowl, combine the rest of the ingredients and blend with a fork. Pour mixture into the pie plate. Bake until golden brown and puffy, about 35 to 45 minutes. Cut into 6 wedges and serve. Serve with 1 cup mixed fruit and 1 cup of fat-free milk. Serves 1.

Nutritional Information: 470 calories; 6g fat (10.8% calories from fat); 21g protein; 87g carbohydrate; 5g dietary fiber; 83mg cholesterol; 590mg sodium.

Lunch

Chicken and Spinach Salad

2 cups cooked chicken, cubed
6 cups packed fresh spinach,
 torn into bite-sized pieces

2 oranges, peeled and cut
 into chunks
2 cups fresh strawberries, sliced

In a large bowl, combine chicken, spinach, oranges and strawberries. Toss with chilled *Orange-Poppy Dressing* (see following recipe) just before serving. Serve each with 6 slices Melba toast. Serves 4.

Orange-Poppy Dressing
2 tbsp. red wine vinegar
3 tbsp. orange juice
$1^1/_2$ tablespoon canola oil
$^1/_4$ tsp. dry mustard
$^1/_4$ tsp. poppy seeds

Combine all and mix well.

Nutritional Information: 307 calories; 9g fat (27.4% calories from fat); 26g protein; 30g carbohydrate; 6g dietary fiber; 60mg cholesterol; 240mg sodium.

Dinner

Wild Rice and Chicken Dinner
1 pkg. long grain and wild rice mix
13-oz. can reduced-fat cream
  of celery soup
$^2/_3$ cup fat-free milk
$^1/_2$ cup reduced-fat mayonnaise
1 tbsp. chopped onion
8-oz. can sliced water
  chestnuts, drained
4 oz. can sliced mushrooms, drained
10-oz. pkg. frozen French-cut
  green beans
1 tbsp. diced fresh rosemary
2 cups diced cooked chicken
$2^1/_2$ cups herb-seasoned
  stuffing mix
1 tbsp. melted margarine
$^1/_2$ cup fat-free chicken broth
nonstick cooking spray

Preheat oven to 350° F. Prepare rice mix according to the directions using water or fat-free chicken broth. Combine soup, milk, mayonnaise, onion, water chestnuts, mushrooms, green beans and rosemary in a bowl. Fold in the chicken. Spray a 9″ x 13″ baking dish with nonstick cooking spray. Combine prepared rice with soup and chicken mixture in the prepared baking dish. In a medium bowl, toss stuffing mix with margarine and broth. Sprinkle over the chicken. Bake for 25 to 30 minutes. Serve with a mixed green salad with light dressing. Serves 8.

Nutritional Information: 376 calories; 9g fat (21.5% calories from fat); 22g protein; 53g carbohydrate; 11g dietary fiber; 35mg cholesterol; 668mg sodium.

DAY 2

Breakfast

1 small (2 oz.) bagel
1 tsp. strawberry all-fruit spread
$^3/_4$ cup light yogurt
$^3/_4$ cup blackberries

Nutritional Information: 318 calories; 2g fat (4.4% calories from fat); 14g protein; 64g carbohydrate; 9g dietary fiber; 2mg cholesterol; 401mg sodium.

Lunch

Stuffed Sweet Potato

(1) 6-oz. baked sweet potato
2 oz. lean ham, diced

1 tsp. reduced-fat margarine
1 tbsp. raisins

Serve with 1 cup steamed asparagus spears drizzled with 1 tablespoon of *Balsamic Vinaigrette* (combine 2 teaspoons balsamic vinegar, 1 teaspoon olive oil and a pinch or garlic powder and mix well). Serves 1.

Nutritional Information: 319 calories; 10g fat (26.7% calories from fat); 16g protein; 44g carbohydrate; 7g dietary fiber; 27mg cholesterol; 876mg sodium.

Dinner

BBQ Steak Kabobs

1¹/₄ lbs. boneless round- or top-
  sirloin steaks, cut into 2-inch pieces
2 tbsp. plus 2 tsp. ketchup
1 tbsp. light molasses
1 tbsp. plus 1 tsp. Worcestershire sauce

2 tsp. spicy brown mustard
2 tsp. grated onion
4 slices French bread, cut ¹/₂-inch
  thick, toasted and hot
1 garlic clove, halved

Preheat grill to medium. In a large bowl, combine ketchup, molasses, Worcestershire sauce, mustard, onion and season with salt (to taste). Add meat; toss to coat well. Thread steak chunks onto long skewers; grill to desired doneness (10 minutes for medium rare), turning occasionally and brushing with sauce. While skewers are cooking, toast the French bread. Lightly rub one side of hot toasted bread with cut side of garlic clove. Serve with 1 cup grilled vegetables and ¹/₂ cup roasted potatoes. Serves 4.

Nutritional Information: 425 calories; 18g fat (38.6% calories from fat); 31g protein; 33g carbohydrate; 2g dietary fiber; 84mg cholesterol; 355mg sodium.

DAY 3

Breakfast

2 lowfat frozen waffles, heated
1 tsp. reduced-calorie margarine
1 tbsp. sugar-free syrup

¹/₂ small mango
1 cup fat-free milk

Nutritional Information: 370 calories; 8g fat (19.2% calories from fat); 13g protein; 63g carbohydrate; 4g dietary fiber; 27mg cholesterol; 727mg sodium.

Lunch

Grilled Turkey and Cheese Sandwich

1¹/₂ oz. sliced cooked turkey breast
2 slices whole-wheat bread
1 tsp. light mayonnaise

1 tsp. mustard
¹/₂-oz. slice Swiss cheese
nonstick cooking spray

Preheat a skillet and coat with nonstick cooking spray. Spread mayonnaise and mustard on bread; layer with turkey and cheese. Grill sandwich over medium heat, turning occasionally, until bread is lightly browned on both sides and cheese is melted. Combine tomato and cucumber in a small bowl; drizzle with dressing prior to serving. Serve with cucumber and tomato salad drizzled with 1 tablespoon *Balsamic Vinaigrette* from yesterday's lunch and one ounce of pretzels. Serves 1.

Nutritional Information: 464 calories; 13g fat (24.9% calories from fat); 29g protein; 62g carbohydrate; 8g dietary fiber; 56mg cholesterol; 978mg sodium.

Dinner

Crockpot Chicken Stew

2 cups water
(4) 4-oz. boneless, skinless chicken
  breasts, cut into chunks
16-oz. low-sodium stewed tomatoes
¹/₂ cup thinly sliced celery
1¹/₂ cups diced carrot
¹/₂ cup chopped onion

¹/₈ tsp. garlic powder
1 bay leaf
¹/₂ tsp. crushed dry leaf basil
¹/₄ tsp. crushed dry leaf oregano
¹/₄ tsp. paprika
1 tsp. low-sodium instant chicken or
  beef bullion

Combine ingredients in a crockpot; cook on low heat for 8 to 10 hours. Discard bay leaf before serving. Serve with a 2-inch cube of cornbread. Serves 4.

Nutritional Information: 524 calories; 11g fat (18.9% calories from fat); 36g protein; 69g carbohydrate; 3g dietary fiber; 118mg cholesterol; 981mg sodium.

DAY 4

Breakfast

Raisin French Toast

1¹/₂ slices cinnamon-raisin bread
¹/₄ cup egg substitute

¹/₄ tsp. vanilla flavoring
1 tbsp. fat-free milk

In a shallow bowl, combine egg substitute, vanilla and milk; add slices of bread, turning until egg mixture is absorbed. Spray a small nonstick skillet or griddle with nonstick cooking spray and preheat. Cook bread over medium heat for 3 to 5 minutes, turning once, until bread is golden brown on both sides. Serve with 1 tablespoon of sugar-free syrup, $1/2$ cup grapefruit sections and $1/2$ cup nonfat milk. Serves 1.

Nutritional Information: 385 calories; 8g fat (18.4% calories from fat); 17g protein; 61g carbohydrate; 3g dietary fiber; 4mg cholesterol; 342mg sodium.

Lunch

Arby's Junior Roast Beef Sandwich®   1 cup green salad with 2 tbsp. light
1 banana   dressing

Nutritional Information: 447 calories; 15g fat (27.9% calories from fat); 20g protein; 65g carbohydrate; 7g dietary fiber; 30mg cholesterol; 794mg sodium.

Dinner

Spaghetti Carbonara
8 oz. uncooked spaghetti noodles   1 cup frozen peas
1 tsp. vegetable oil   1 oz. freshly grated Parmesan cheese
1 medium onion, chopped   2 tbsp. reduced-fat sour cream
$2/3$ cup reduced-sodium chicken broth   freshly ground black pepper
3 cups sliced mushrooms   additional Parmesan cheese for
8 oz. lean Canadian bacon, thinly   garnish (optional)
   sliced into strips   nonstick cooking spray

Cook spaghetti noodles according to package directions, omitting salt and fat, and drain. Return noodles to the pot and toss with oil to prevent sticking. Set aside. Coat a large skillet with nonstick cooking spray. Sauté onion over medium-high heat until tender. Add broth and bring to a boil. Add mushrooms and cook 4 to 5 minutes, stirring frequently. Add bacon strips. Cook for an additional 2 to 3 minutes; add peas. When heated through, remove from heat. Stir in cheese and sour cream. Garnish each serving with pepper and fresh Parmesan. Serve with 1 cup green salad, 2 tablespoons lowfat dressing and a 1-ounce slice of toasted French bread. Serves 4.

Nutritional Information: 543 calories; 10g fat (17.4% calories from fat); 31g protein; 80g carbohydrate; 6g dietary fiber; 34mg cholesterol; 1,415mg sodium.

DAY 5

Breakfast

$^1/_2$ large bagel, toasted
2 tbsp. fat-free cream cheese

1 small orange
1 cup fat-free milk

Nutritional Information: 335 calories; 6g fat (16.7% calories from fat); 17g protein; 53g carbohydrate; 4g dietary fiber; 20mg cholesterol; 523mg sodium.

Lunch

Grilled Turkey Burger

2 oz. grilled ground turkey
1 slice light American cheese
2 oz. hamburger roll

1 cup tomato
1 cup Spanish onion slices
2 iceberg lettuce leaves

Serve burger with Russian dressing (combine $2^1/_2$ teaspoons light mayonnaise and ketchup in a cup or a small bowl) and *Oven Fries* (see following recipe). Serves 1.

Nutritional Information: 492 calories; 19g fat (34% calories from fat); 26g protein; 57g carbohydrate; 7g dietary fiber; 68mg cholesterol; 996mg sodium.

Oven Fries

(1) 3-oz. baking potato, cut into
  thin sticks
$^1/_4$ tsp. salt

$^1/_4$ tsp. paprika
nonstick cooking spray

Preheat oven to 450° F. Place potato sticks onto a nonstick baking sheet and spray them lightly with nonstick cooking spray. Sprinkle with salt and paprika and bake for 10 to 12 minutes or until crispy outside and tender inside. Serves 1.

Nutritional Information: 69 calories; trace fat (2% calories from fat); 2g protein; 16g carbohydrate; 1g dietary fiber; 0mg cholesterol; 538mg sodium.

Dinner

Seafood Restaurant Dinner

broiled or grilled seafood entrée
  (sauce on the side)
$^1/_2$ cup rice

$^1/_2$ cup steamed or grilled vegetables
2 cups salad
2 tbsp. low-fat dressing (on the side)

Nutritional Information: 508 calories; 8g fat (15% calories from fat); 24g protein; 81g carbohydrate; 5g dietary fiber; 49mg cholesterol; 549mg sodium.

DAY 6

....

Breakfast

Potato Omelet

1 potato, unpeeled	6 eggs, well beaten, or 1$^1/_2$ cups
1 tbsp. olive oil	liquid egg substitute
1 medium onion, sliced thin	4-oz. can chopped green chilies
1 tsp. minced garlic	

Preheat oven to 350° F. Poke the potato with a fork several times and microwave on high power for 5 minutes or until tender. Cut the potato into thin slices. In an 8-inch oven-proof skillet, sauté onion and garlic in olive oil for 3 minutes. Remove from heat, pour eggs into the skillet and sprinkle chilies and potato slices on top. Bake for 10 to 12 minutes or until the egg is well set. Use a spatula to carefully fold omelet in half. Cut into 4 wedges and serve with 1 cup of strawberries with two tablespoons of Cool Whip Lite®. Serves 4.

Nutritional Information: 371 calories; 19g fat (47.1% calories from fat); 12g protein; 35g carbohydrate; 5g dietary fiber; 318mg cholesterol; 153mg sodium.

....

Lunch

Tortellini Soup

$^1/_2$ cup chopped onion	1 tsp. sugar
46-oz. can vegetable juice	$^1/_4$ tsp. seasoned salt
2 cups water	$^1/_2$ tsp. oregano
2 no-added-salt chicken bouillon	$^1/_2$ tsp. basil
cubes	8-oz. pkg. dry tortellini with
10-oz. pkg. frozen spinach	Parmesan cheese
2 carrots, chopped	nonstick cooking spray

Sauté onion in a nonstick skillet that has been sprayed with nonstick cooking spray. Add vegetable juice, water, bouillon, frozen block of spinach, carrots, sugar, salt and seasonings. Bring to a boil. Turn heat to medium and simmer for 15 minutes. Bring to a boil again and add tortellini. Simmer for another 30 minutes. Serves 8. Serve with 3-inch slice French bread and 1 cup mixed fruit.

Nutritional Information: 498 calories; 5g fat (8.3% calories from fat); 15g protein; 102g carbohydrate; 9g dietary fiber; 39mg cholesterol; 785mg sodium.

Dinner

Chicken Fajita

1¹/₂ oz. cooked chicken, shredded
¹/₄ cup onion, diced
¹/₄ cup bell pepper, diced
¹/₄ cup salsa

1 tbsp. fat-free sour cream
(1) 10-inch lowfat flour tortilla
¹/₄ oz. Colby cheese, shredded
nonstick cooking spray

In skillet coated with cooking spray, sauté onions and peppers for 1 minute; add chicken and heat thoroughly. In a small bowl, combine salsa and sour cream; mix well. Fill tortilla with chicken and top with cheese. Heat in microwave, if desired, and serve with creamy salsa. Serve with 1 cup canned tropical mixed fruit. Serves 1.

Nutritional Information: 393 calories; 6g fat (13.8% calories from fat); 19g protein; 66g carbohydrate; 8g dietary fiber; 44mg cholesterol; 709mg sodium.

DAY 7

Breakfast

1 slice cinnamon-raisin bread, toasted
1 tsp. reduced-calorie margarine
¹/₂ tsp. granulated sugar

pinch of cinnamon
³/₄ cup plain nonfat yogurt
³/₄ cup blueberries

Nutritional Information: 281 calories; 3g fat (9.7% calories from fat); 14g protein; 51g carbohydrate; 4g dietary fiber; 3mg cholesterol; 283mg sodium.

Lunch

Asiago and Asparagus Omelet

3 stalks asparagus
2 eggs
2 tbsp. water

salt and fresh ground pepper (to taste)
1 oz. sliced Asiago cheese
pinch of fresh tarragon

Chop the asparagus stalks, leaving the tops for ornamentation. Steam the chopped stalks until tender (about 4 to 8 minutes). Heat a nonstick pan that has been brushed with oil. Whisk together eggs, water, salt and pepper. Pour egg mixture into pan, swirling around and lifting gently so that all eggs cook. While eggs are cooking, place the steamed asparagus and cheese on half of the omelet. Sprinkle with tarragon. Gently fold the other half over. Once set, lift and move omelet to serve or keep in warm oven until all omelets are ready. Arrange reserved asparagus tops in a semi-circle and lay a tarragon twig on top. Serve with 1/2 cup grapes. Serves 1.

Nutritional Information: 292 calories; 18g fat (55.6% calories from fat); 21g protein; 12g carbohydrate; 1g dietary fiber; 449mg cholesterol; 489mg sodium.

....

Dinner

Mexican Chicken

10 oz. boneless, skinless chicken breasts, cooked and diced
(12) 6-inch corn tortillas, torn into pieces
(2) 10-oz. cans reduced-fat cream of chicken soup
(1) 10-oz. can rotel tomatoes
8 oz. Velveeta® light processed cheese
1 bell pepper, chopped
1 onion, chopped
nonstick cooking spray

Preheat oven to 350° F. In a medium saucepan, heat soup, tomatoes and cheese until cheese is melted. Sauté bell pepper and onion in nonstick skillet with 1/4 cup of water or broth until tender. Stir into soup mixture; add chicken and tortillas. Pour into 9" x 13" baking dish coated with nonstick cooking spray. Bake for 30 minutes. Serve with 2 cups mixed greens with light ranch dressing. (Add a little cumin or chopped jalapeno to your low-fat dressing to spice it up!) Serves 8.

Nutritional Information: 272 calories; 7g fat (24.9% calories from fat); 23g protein; 26g carbohydrate; 4g dietary fiber; 38mg cholesterol; 989mg sodium.

Second Week Grocery List

Produce
- [ ] apples
- [ ] apricots
- [ ] asparagus
- [ ] baby carrots
- [ ] baby spinach
- [ ] bananas
- [ ] basil
- [ ] blackberries
- [ ] blueberries
- [ ] broccoli
- [ ] broccoli slaw mix (1 bag)
- [ ] carrots
- [ ] cherry tomatoes
- [ ] corn on the cob
- [ ] garlic cloves
- [ ] ginger, fresh
- [ ] grapes, seedless
- [ ] grapefruit
- [ ] green beans
- [ ] green bell pepper
- [ ] green scallions
- [ ] kiwi fruit
- [ ] lemon
- [ ] lettuce
- [ ] limes
- [ ] mushrooms
- [ ] nectarines
- [ ] olives
- [ ] onions
- [ ] oranges
- [ ] parsley
- [ ] peaches
- [ ] potatoes
- [ ] red bell peppers
- [ ] red grapes
- [ ] red onion
- [ ] snap peas
- [ ] strawberries
- [ ] sweet cherries
- [ ] tomatoes
- [ ] white scallions

Baking Products
- [ ] all-fruit spread
- [ ] almonds, slivered
- [ ] apricot preserves
- [ ] artificial sweetener
- [ ] baking powder
- [ ] bay leaves
- [ ] black pepper
- [ ] brown mustard
- [ ] brown rice, instant
- [ ] brown sugar
- [ ] Caesar dressing, light
- [ ] canola oil
- [ ] cayenne pepper
- [ ] celery seed
- [ ] cooking oil
- [ ] cornstarch
- [ ] couscous
- [ ] dressing, lowfat
- [ ] dry mustard
- [ ] fig preserves
- [ ] flour, all-purpose
- [ ] flour, whole-wheat
- [ ] honey
- [ ] Italian herb seasoning
- [ ] ketchup
- [ ] lemon juice
- [ ] marmalade, orange
- [ ] nonstick cooking spray
- [ ] oats, quick-cooking
- [ ] olive oil

- ❑ oregano, dried
- ❑ parsley
- ❑ peanut butter
- ❑ pecans, chopped
- ❑ pepper
- ❑ powdered sugar
- ❑ ranch dressing, light
- ❑ red pepper flakes
- ❑ rice
- ❑ salsa
- ❑ salt
- ❑ soy sauce
- ❑ sugar
- ❑ sweet pickle relish
- ❑ Tabasco sauce
- ❑ tarragon
- ❑ thyme, dried
- ❑ white vinegar

Breads and Cereals

- ❑ bread, cinnamon-raisin
- ❑ bread, whole-wheat
- ❑ bread crumbs
- ❑ dinner roll
- ❑ English muffins
- ❑ French bread
- ❑ pitas, whole-wheat
- ❑ rotini
- ❑ saltine crackers
- ❑ spaghetti
- ❑ tortillas, whole-wheat
- ❑ tostada shells

Canned Foods

- ❑ chicken broth
- ❑ 15 oz. Italian-style tomatoes, diced (1 can)
- ❑ 12 oz. refried beans (1 can)
- ❑ 1 lb. tomatoes (1 can)
- ❑ 1 lb., 14 oz. tomatoes (1 can)
- ❑ tuna, light

Dairy Products

- ❑ buttermilk, lowfat
- ❑ cheddar cheese, reduced-fat
- ❑ eggs
- ❑ egg substitute
- ❑ goat cheese
- ❑ half-and-half, fat-free
- ❑ margarine, light
- ❑ mayonnaise, lowfat
- ❑ milk, fat-free
- ❑ Mozzarella cheese
- ❑ Parmesan cheese
- ❑ sour cream, nonfat
- ❑ white grape juice

Frozen Foods

- ❑ hash browns, shredded
- ❑ Lean Cuisine Chicken Club Panini®
- ❑ vegetables (broccoli, cauliflower, carrots)
- ❑ waffles, whole-wheat

Meat and Poultry

- ❑ chicken breasts (with bones and skin)
- ❑ chicken breasts, boneless, skinless
- ❑ ground beef
- ❑ halibut fillets ($1^1/_4$ lbs.)
- ❑ ham, lean
- ❑ turkey breakfast sausage, light

Second Week Meals and Recipes

DAY 1

Breakfast

Oatmeal Nut Waffles

1¹/₂ cup whole-wheat flour
2 tsp. baking powder
¹/₂ tsp. salt
2 eggs, lightly beaten
2 cups fat-free milk

2 tbsp. margarine, melted
2 tbsp. nonfat sour cream
2 tbsp. honey
1 cup quick-cooking oats
2 tbsp. chopped pecans

In a mixing bowl, combine flour, baking powder and salt. In a separate small mixing bowl, combine eggs, milk, margarine, sour cream and honey. Stir liquid into dry ingredients and mix well. Fold in oats and nuts. Preheat a waffle iron and cook the waffles. Serve with 1 cup of fresh peaches. Serves 1.

Nutritional Information: 358 calories; 7g fat (19.9% calories from fat); 11g protein; 69g carbohydrate; 10g dietary fiber; 55mg cholesterol; 342mg sodium.

Lunch

Spicy Thai Chicken

(2) 4-oz. boneless, skinless chicken
  breasts
1 small red bell pepper, chopped
2 tbsp. white vinegar

¹/₄ tsp. red pepper flakes, crushed
1 tsp. sugar
1 lime sliced into 6 wedges
artificial sweetener

In a food processor, puree red bell pepper with vinegar and pour puree into a saucepan. Add red pepper flakes and bring to a boil. Reduce heat and simmer for 3 minutes. Remove from heat. Once cooled, stir in artificial sweetener. Broil chicken breasts in a preheated oven for 10 minutes or until browned, and then turn pieces and broil approximately 5 minutes more. While broiling chicken, prepare serving platter with a bed of hot cooked white or brown rice or couscous. Remove chicken from the oven and place on the bed of rice/couscous. Spoon sauce over the chicken, garnish with lime wedges, and serve immediately. Serve each with ²/₃ cup rice or couscous and ¹/₂ cup sautéed snap peas. Serves 2.

Nutritional Information: 621 calories; 2g fat (3.4% calories from fat); 43g protein; 104g carbohydrate; 9g dietary fiber; 66mg cholesterol; 91mg sodium.

Dinner

Chicken Supreme with Mushroom Gravy

(6) 3-oz. boneless, skinless chicken
  breasts
1 cup bread crumbs
1 cup grated Parmesan cheese
1 tsp. salt

$1/4$ tsp. black pepper
2 tbsp. parsley
1 garlic clove, minced
$1/4$ oz. slivered almonds
3 egg whites

Preheat oven to 350° F. Slightly beat egg whites in a small bowl and set aside. Combine bread crumbs, cheese, salt, pepper, parsley, garlic and almonds (reserve a few for garnish) in a shallow dish. Dip chicken breasts in egg whites, roll in bread crumb mixture, and arrange in 9" x 13" baking dish. Garnish with a few almond slivers. Bake for 30 minutes. Serve each with 1 cup of green beans and an ear of corn on the cob. Serves 6.

Nutritional Information: 354 calories; 8g fat (25.5% calories from fat); 34g protein; 39g carbohydrate; 7g dietary fiber; 60mg cholesterol; 862mg sodium.

Mushroom Gravy

$1/4$ cup light margarine
2 cups sliced mushrooms
1 cup chicken broth

2 tsp. cornstarch
1 tsp. salt
pepper (to taste)

Sauté mushrooms in melted margarine. Gradually add broth to the mixture in the skillet and continue to stir. Dissolve cornstarch in a small amount of liquid. Add to the skillet mixture, stirring constantly until thickened. Add seasonings to taste. Spoon over the chicken breasts and serve. Serves 6.

Nutritional Information: 49 calories; 4g fat (72.7% calories from fat); 1g protein; 2g carbohydrate; trace dietary fiber; 0mg cholesterol; 575mg sodium.

DAY TWO

Breakfast

Breakfast Sammy

1 whole-grain English muffin
1 oz. reduced-fat cheddar cheese

$1^1/2$ oz. light turkey breakfast
  sausage

Assemble and serve with 1 orange. Serves 1.

Nutritional Information: 300 calories; 12g fat (4g saturated fat); 21g protein; 28g carbohydrate; 5g fiber; 83mg cholesterol; 690mg sodium.

Lunch

1 whole-wheat pita	1 lettuce leaf
2 oz. cooked chicken breast, cubed	light Caesar dressing

Assemble pita sandwich and serve with 1 cup baby carrots and an apple. Serves 1.

Nutritional Information: 433 calories; 7g fat (13.7% calories from fat); 22g protein; 76g carbohydrate; 13g dietary fiber; 39mg cholesterol; 457mg sodium.

Dinner

Chicken and Bean Tostadas

8 tostada shells	8 oz. shredded reduced-fat cheddar
8 oz. cooked chicken breast, cubed	cheese
(1) 12-oz. can fat-free refried beans	1 cup chopped tomato
1 cup shredded lettuce	salsa

Preheat oven to 350° F. Spread a thin layer of refried beans on each shell and place on a cookie sheet. Sprinkle 2 ounces of cheddar cheese on each shell. Add 1 ounce of cooked chicken to each shell. Bake in the oven for 7 to 10 minutes until beans are warmed and shell is crispy. Add lettuce, tomato and salsa as desired. Serves 4.

Nutritional Information: 456 calories; 18g fat (36% calories from fat); 27g protein; 46g carbohydrate; 6g dietary fiber; 45mg cholesterol; 629mg sodium.

DAY 3

Breakfast

2 slices whole-wheat bread	$1/2$ medium grapefruit
1 tbsp. peanut butter	1 cup fat-free milk

Nutritional Information: 357 calories; 11g fat (26.6% calories from fat); 19g protein; 50g carbohydrate; 6g dietary fiber; 4mg cholesterol; 497mg sodium.

Lunch

Wendy's Ultimate Chicken Grill Sandwich® and Mandarin Orange Cup

Nutritional Information: 402 calories; 8g fat (17.2% calories from fat); 29g protein; 59g carbohydrate; 4g dietary fiber; 65mg cholesterol; 802mg sodium.

Dinner

Chicken Breasts with Asparagus and Carrots

(4) 4-oz. boneless, skinless
  chicken breasts, cut crosswise into
  $1/4$-inch strips
$1/2$ lb. fresh asparagus spears,
  trimmed and cut into 1-inch lengths
2 medium carrots, cut into $1/8$-inch
  thick rounds

1 small onion, thinly sliced
2 tbsp. reduced-fat margarine,
  melted
2 tsp. lemon juice
$1/2$ tsp. tarragon
$1/8$ tsp. cayenne pepper
salt and pepper (to taste)

Preheat oven to 450° F. Tear off a large piece of aluminum foil for each serving. Arrange chicken in the center of the lower half of each piece of foil. Season with salt and pepper and top with equal amounts of asparagus, carrot and onion. In a small bowl, combine melted margarine, lemon juice, tarragon, cayenne pepper and salt. Pour equal amounts of the liquid over each serving of chicken. For each serving, fold two ends of foil together tightly three or four times. Repeat process with ends to seal packet tightly. Arrange foil packets in a single layer on the baking sheet. Bake 20 minutes and serve. Serve each with 1-ounce dinner roll and $1/2$ cup cooked rice. Serves 4.

Nutritional Information: 389 calories; 7g fat (15.8% calories from fat); 33g protein; 48g carbohydrate; 3g dietary fiber; 66mg cholesterol; 306mg sodium.

DAY 4

Breakfast

Veggie Microwave Frittata

$1^1/4$ cups shredded frozen hash
  browns (the type with no fat
  grams per serving)
$2/3$ cup shredded or grated carrot
$1/4$ cup chopped onion
1 tbsp. chopped fresh parsley
  (or $1^1/2$ tsp. parsley flakes)
2 tsp. olive oil or canola oil
$1/2$ cup egg substitute

2 large eggs (use a higher omega-3
  brand if available)
$1/4$ cup lowfat milk or fat-free half-
  and-half
$1/8$ tsp. dry mustard
two dashes hot pepper sauce
$1/2$ cup shredded reduced-fat sharp
  cheddar cheese
pinch of salt and pepper (optional)

In a microwave-safe 1-quart casserole dish, combine potatoes, carrot, onion, parsley and oil. Cover and microwave on high for 3 minutes, stirring after 90 seconds. Add salt and pepper, if desired. In a mixing bowl, combine eggs, egg substitute, milk, mustard and hot pepper sauce by beating on medium speed for a minute or two. Pour egg mixture into a casserole dish and stir to combine with potato mixture. Cover dish (waxed paper will work) and microwave on high for 2 minutes. Draw cooked egg toward the middle of the dish and the liquid egg toward the edges and microwave on high for 2 minutes more. Sprinkle cheese on top and microwave until cheese is melted (about 30 seconds more). Let stand a few minutes before serving. Serve each with 1 cup fresh fruit. Serves 3.

Nutritional Information: 313 calories; 13g fat (37.4% calories from fat); 17g protein; 33g carbohydrate; 6g dietary fiber; 146mg cholesterol; 284mg sodium.

Lunch

Lean Cuisine Chicken Club Panini®

1 1/2 cups frozen vegetables (broccoli, cauliflower, carrots)

Nutritional Information: 320 calories; 7g fat (18.4% calories from fat); 18g protein; 49g carbohydrate; 10g dietary fiber; 40mg cholesterol; 656mg sodium.

Dinner

Garlic and Ginger Braised Halibut Fillets

1 1/4 lbs. 1-inch thick halibut fillets cut into 4 pieces
1 small onion, minced
2 white scallions, chopped
2 green scallions, chopped into 1-inch lengths
3 garlic cloves, minced

2 tbsp. minced fresh ginger
1/8 tsp. red pepper flakes, crushed
1/4 cup white grape juice
1/2 cup canned chicken broth
2 cups instant brown rice, uncooked
nonstick cooking spray

Lightly coat a large nonstick skillet with nonstick cooking spray. Preheat until very hot, but not smoking. Add fillets and brown them skin side down for 2 minutes. Add onion, scallions, garlic, ginger and red pepper flakes. Cook on high for 1 minute. Reduce heat and turn fillets. Add grape juice and broth; cover pan and simmer for 10 minutes or until cooked through. (Insert a small, thick knife into the fish to check if it is done.) While fish is simmering, prepare 4 servings of instant brown rice according to package directions. Serve the fish over rice and spoon some of the sauce over the fillets. Serve each with 1 cup *Broccoli Slaw* (see following recipe) and 2/3 cup rice. Serves 4.

Nutritional Information: 432 calories; 4g fat (7.4% calories from fat); 35g protein; 63g carbohydrate; 4g dietary fiber; 45mg cholesterol; 200mg sodium.

Broccoli Slaw

(1) 16-oz. bag shredded broccoli slaw mix	1 tsp. prepared brown mustard
$1/4$ cup sweet pickle relish	$1/4$ tsp. celery seed
$1/3$ cup lowfat mayonnaise	$1/4$ tsp. black pepper
	1 cup (about 15) red grapes (optional)

Combine all ingredients in large bowl; refrigerate until needed. Serves 4.

Nutritional Information: 161 calories; 7g fat (35.4% calories from fat); 2g protein; 27g carbohydrate; 2g dietary fiber; 16mg cholesterol; 267mg sodium.

DAY 5

Breakfast

Fruit-filled Pancakes

1 whole egg plus 1 egg white	$1/4$ tsp. salt
$1/4$ cup all-purpose flour	2 cups fresh fruit
$1/4$ cup fat-free milk	2 tbsp. orange marmalade, warmed
1 tbsp. cooking oil	nonstick cooking spray

Coat four $4^1/4$-inch pie plates or $4^1/2$-inch foil tart pans with nonstick cooking spray and set aside. In a mixing bowl, use a rotary beater or wire whisk to beat whole egg, egg white, flour, milk, oil and salt until smooth. Divide batter among prepared pans. Bake at 400° F for about 25 minutes or until brown and puffy. Turn off oven and let pancakes stand in oven for 5 minutes. To serve, immediately transfer the pancakes from the oven to 4 plates. Spoon some of the fruit (choose from sliced strawberries, peeled and sliced kiwi fruit or peaches, blackberries, blueberries, seedless grapes, sliced nectarines or apricots and/or pitted and halved sweet cherries) into the center of each pancake. Drizzle fruit with warmed orange marmalade. Serves 4.

Nutritional Information: 123 calories; 4g fat; 1g saturated fat; 5g protein; 18g carbohydrate; 2g dietary fiber; 213 mg cholesterol; 210mg sodium.

Lunch

3 oz. light tuna, drained	$1/2$ cup diced tomatoes
2 tbsp. fresh parsley, chopped	dash of salt and pepper
$1/2$ lemon, juiced	2 whole-grain tortillas
1 tbsp. olive oil	$1/2$ cup baby spinach

Combine tuna with parsley, lemon, oil, tomatoes, salt and pepper. Wrap the mixture in the tortillas and top with spinach. Serve each with 1 cup mixed fruit. Serves 2.

Nutritional Information: 309 calories; 10g fat (28.9% calories from fat); 17g protein; 40g carbohydrate; 6g dietary fiber; 13mg cholesterol; 538mg sodium.

Dinner
BBQ Chicken Breasts with Apricot Glaze

4 chicken breast halves (about
   1¹/₂ lbs.) with skin on and bone in
¹/₃ cup apricot preserves
1 tbsp. soy sauce

1 tbsp. water
2 tbsp. plus 2 tsp. ketchup
2 tsp. brown sugar

Preheat grill to medium. Grill chicken (with skin on) for 10 minutes, turning occasionally. Remove from the grill and remove the skin. In a small bowl, combine preserves, soy sauce, water, ketchup and brown sugar. Blend well. Return chicken to the grill and generously brush with glaze. Continue cooking for 10 to 15 minutes or until thoroughly done, turning often and brushing with glaze frequently. Serve each with 1 cup mashed potatoes and 1 cup seasoned green beans. Serves 4.

Nutritional Information: 515 calories; 17g fat (30% calories from fat); 35g protein; 56g carbohydrate; 8g dietary fiber; 91mg cholesterol; 941mg sodium.

DAY 6

Breakfast
PB&J Waffle Sandwich

2 whole-wheat frozen waffles
1 tbsp. peanut butter

2 tsp. all-fruit spread

Assemble sandwich and serve with 1 banana. Serves 1.

Nutritional Information: 299 calories; 14g fat (40.5% calories from fat); 8g protein; 37g carbohydrate; 2g dietary fiber; 22mg cholesterol; 601mg sodium.

Lunch

Creamy Pasta Salad

3 cups cooked rotini (corkscrew
   pasta)

1 cup broccoli florets
1 cup quartered cherry tomatoes

3/4 cup diced lean ham (3 oz.)
1/2 cup sliced carrot
1/2 cup vertically sliced red onion
1/3 cup sliced ripe olives
1/4 cup grated Parmesan cheese
1/4 cup light ranch dressing

2 tbsp. chopped fresh or 2 tsp.
  dried basil
2 tbsp. chopped fresh parsley or
  2 tsp. dried parsley flakes
1/4 cup fat-free sour cream
1/4 cup low-fat buttermilk

Combine rotini, broccoli, cherry tomatoes, ham, carrot, red onion, olives, Parmesan cheese, basil and parsley in a bowl. Combine sour cream, buttermilk and dressing and stir well. Pour over salad and toss to coat. Serve each with 6 saltine crackers. Serves 4.

Nutritional Information: 296 calories; 5g fat (16.2% calories from fat); 13g protein; 48g carbohydrate; 3g dietary fiber; 12mg cholesterol; 597mg sodium.

....

Dinner

Chicken Cacciatore Pie

1 lb. ground chicken breast
(1) 15-oz. can Italian-style diced
  tomatoes, drained (reserve
  3 1/2 tbsp. juice)
3/4 small onion, chopped
3/4 small green bell pepper, chopped
garlic clove, minced

1/3 cup plain bread crumbs
egg
1 1/4 tsp. Italian herb seasoning
1/3 cup fat-free Mozzarella cheese,
  shredded
2 tbsp. Parmesan cheese, grated

Preheat oven to 350° F. In a medium bowl, combine reserved tomato juice, onion, bell pepper, garlic, bread crumbs and egg. Add half the Italian seasoning, salt and pepper (to taste). Mix thoroughly. Add ground chicken and mix well. Pat mixture evenly into a lightly oiled 10-inch pie plate, pushing up the sides to form a shell. Bake for 25 minutes. In a stainless steel sauce-pan, combine tomatoes, remaining Italian seasoning and salt and pepper to taste. Simmer for 10 to 15 minutes over medium heat, and then remove from heat and set aside. Remove meat shell from the oven and discard excess liquid. Sprinkle the shell with mozzarella cheese. Add tomato sauce, sprinkle with Parmesan cheese, and bake for 15 minutes until meat shell is cooked throughout. Let stand for 5 minutes before cutting and serving. Serve each with 1 cup green salad, 2 tablespoons lowfat dressing and a 1-ounce slice of toasted French bread. Serves 4.

Nutritional Information: 348 calories; 18g fat (46% calories from fat); 12g protein; 34g carbohydrate; 5g dietary fiber; 57mg cholesterol; 940mg sodium.

DAY 7

Breakfast

McDonald's Egg McMuffin® without cheese   apple dippers

Nutritional Information: 390 calories; 9g fat; 17g protein; 62g carbohydrate; 2g dietary fiber; 245mg cholesterol; 585mg sodium.

Lunch

Grilled Goat Cheese Sandwich

2 tsp. honey
$1/4$ tsp. grated lemon rind
(1) 4-oz. pkg. goat cheese
(8) 1-oz. slices cinnamon-raisin
  bread
2 tbsp. fig preserves

2 tsp. thinly sliced fresh basil
1 tsp. powdered sugar
nonstick cooking spray

Combine honey, lemon rind and goat cheese, stirring until well blended. Spread 1 tablespoon of goat cheese mixture on each of 4 bread slices; top each slice with $1^1/_2$ teaspoons preserves and $1/_2$ teaspoon basil. Top with remaining bread slices. Lightly coat the outside of the bread with nonstick cooking spray. Heat a large nonstick skillet over medium heat. Add 2 sandwiches to the pan. Place a cast-iron or heavy skillet on top of the sandwiches and press gently to flatten. Cook for 3 minutes on each side or until bread is lightly toasted. (Leave the cast-iron skillet on sandwiches while they cook.) Repeat with remaining sandwiches. Sprinkle with sugar. Serves 4.

Nutritional Information: 288 calories; 11g fat (34.3% calories from fat); 13g protein; 34g carbohydrate; 2g dietary fiber; 30mg cholesterol; 240mg sodium.

Dinner

Spaghetti with Meat Sauce

1 cup chopped onion
1 lb. ground beef
2 cloves garlic, minced

(1) 1-lb., 14-oz. can tomatoes,
  cut up
(1) 6-oz. can tomato paste

¹/₄ cup snipped parsley
1 tbsp. brown sugar
1 tsp. salt
1¹/₂ tsp. dried oregano, crushed

¹/₄ tsp. dried thyme, crushed
1 bay leaf
hot cooked spaghetti
Parmesan cheese

In a Dutch oven, combine onion, meat and garlic. Cook until the meat is browned and onion is tender. Skim off excess fat. Add tomatoes, tomato paste, parsley, brown sugar, salt, oregano and thyme and 2 cups of water. Simmer, uncovered, for 3 hours or until sauce is thick, stirring occasionally. Remove bay leaf. Serve over hot spaghetti. Pass around a bowl of shredded Parmesan cheese. Serves 6.

Nutritional Information: 464 calories; 22g fat (41.5% calories from fat); 21g protein; 48g carbohydrate; 5g dietary fiber; 64mg cholesterol; 595mg sodium.

DESSERT AND SNACK RECIPES

(**Note:** You will need to add the ingredients for each of these items to the grocery lists.)

Orange Julius
6-oz. can frozen orange juice
1 cup fat-free milk
¹/₄ cup sugar

1 cup water
1 tsp. vanilla
12 ice cubes

Place all ingredients in a blender. Process until slushy. Serves 6.

Nutritional Information: 94 calories; trace fat (1.3% calories from fat); 2g protein; 21g carbohydrate; trace dietary fiber; 1mg cholesterol; 24mg sodium.

Frosty Orange Cup
10 large oranges
(2) 16-oz. cans apricot halves with
  juice, chopped
10¹/₂-oz. can pineapple tidbits with
  juice
3 bananas, sliced

1 cup flaked coconut
¹/₂ cup sugar
6-oz. frozen orange juice
  concentrate, thawed
1 tbsp. fresh lemon juice

Cut each orange in half. Remove orange sections and reserve. Place orange shells in the freezer until thoroughly chilled. Combine orange sections with remaining ingredients and mix thoroughly. Spoon the mixture into prepared orange shells. Return to the freezer for at least 3 hours. Remove from the freezer 30 minutes before serving. Extra orange mixture may be frozen in muffin tins lined with paper baking cups. Serves 20.

Nutritional Information: 116 calories; 1g fat (6.3% calories from fat); 2g protein; 32g carbohydrate; 4g dietary fiber; 0mg cholesterol; 13mg sodium.

Fruity Salad with Marshmallows

16-oz. can fruit cocktail in juice, drained
2 bananas, sliced
1 pint fresh raspberries or strawberries, sliced

1 cup mini marshmallows
1 cup nonfat strawberry or raspberry yogurt
2 cups nonfat whipped topping

Fold all ingredients together gently and chill. Serves 20.

Nutritional Information: 91 calories; 2g fat (15.4% calories from fat); 1g protein; 18g carbohydrate; 2g dietary fiber; trace cholesterol; 22mg sodium.

Fruit with Yogurt Dressing

(1) 8-oz. container sugar-free fat-free yogurt

(1) 16-oz. container Cool Whip Lite®

Serve over fruit. Serves 16 (2-tablespoon) servings.

Nutritional Information (for dressing only): 78 calories; 4g fat (47.5% calories from fat); 1g protein; 8g carbohydrate; trace dietary fiber; trace cholesterol; 29mg sodium.

Pita Pizza

2 medium pita breads (about 6 inches)
4 minced garlic cloves
bunch of fresh basil

2 sliced tomatoes
1/2 cup shredded Mozzarella cheese
2 tsp. extra virgin olive oil

Preheat oven to 400° F. Separate each pita into two parts. Put the pita bread on cookie sheets. Spread 1 minced garlic clove onto each pita round. Arrange 4 to 6 basil leaves over the garlic. Top with 3 slices of tomato. Sprinkle about 2 tablespoons of shredded Mozzarella cheese on each and drizzle with olive oil. Bake for about 15 minutes or until the cheese melts and the pizzas are bubbly. Serve as whole pizza immediately.

Nutritional Information: 154 calories; 6g fat (36% calories from fat); 6g protein; 19g carbo-hydrate; 1g dietary fiber; 13mg cholesterol; 221mg sodium.

Double Layered Chocolate Pie

$1^1/_2$ cups cold fat-free milk plus
  1 tbsp. milk
(2) 4-serving size chocolate-flavored
  sugar-free instant puddings

4 oz. fat-free cream cheese, softened
1 pkg. sweetener
4 oz. Cool Whip Lite®, thawed
1 reduced-fat graham cracker crust

Pour $1^1/_2$ cups milk into medium bowl and add pudding mix. Beat with an electric mixer for one minute (mixture will be very thick). Spread mixture evenly into piecrust. Beat cream cheese, sweetener, and 1 tablespoon of milk with mixer until smooth. Fold in Cool Whip Lite® on low-speed. Spread over chocolate mixture. Cover and chill at least three hours before serving. Serves 8.

Nutritional Information: 186 calories; 6g fat (28.5% calories from fat); 5g protein; 27g car-bohydrate; 1g dietary fiber; 2mg cholesterol; 327mg sodium.

Member Survey

Please answer the following questions to help your leader plan your First Place 4 Health meetings so that your needs might be met in this session. Give this form to your leader at the first group meeting.

Name _____   Birth date _____

Please list those who live in your household.

Name	Relationship	Age
_____	_____	_____
_____	_____	_____
_____	_____	_____
_____	_____	_____

What church do you attend? _____

Are you interested in receiving more information about our church?

      Yes   No

Occupation _____

What talent or area of expertise would you be willing to share with our class?

_____

Why did you join First Place 4 Health?

_____

With notice, would you be willing to lead a Bible study discussion one week?

      Yes   No

Are you comfortable praying out loud? _____

If the assistant leader were absent, would you be willing to assist in weighing in members and possibly evaluating the Live It Trackers?

      Yes   No

Any other comments:

_____

_____

Personal Weight and Measurement Record

Week	Weight	+ or -	Goal this Session	Pounds to goal
1				
2				
3				
4				
5				
6				
7				
8				
9				
10				
11				
12				

Beginning Measurements

Waist _____ Hips _____ Thighs _____ Chest _____

Ending Measurements

Waist _____ Hips _____ Thighs _____ Chest _____

First Place 4 Health
Prayer Partner

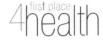

SCRIPTURE VERSE TO MEMORIZE FOR WEEK TWO:

But God demonstrates his own love for us in this:
While we were still sinners, Christ died for us.

ROMANS 5:8

Date: _____

Name: _____

Home Phone: (_____) _____

Work Phone: (_____) _____

Email: _____

Personal Prayer Concerns:

_____

_____

_____

_____

_____

_____

_____

This form is for prayer requests that are personal to you and your journey in First Place 4 Health. Please complete this form and have it ready to turn in when you arrive at your group meeting.

First Place 4 Health
Prayer Partner

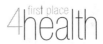

GROWING IN THE
FRUIT OF THE SPIRIT
Week
2

SCRIPTURE VERSE TO MEMORIZE FOR WEEK THREE:

"For I know the plans I have for you," declares the LORD, "plans to prosper you and not to harm you, plans to give you hope and a future."

JEREMIAH 29:11

Date: _____

Name: _____

Home Phone: (_____) _____

Work Phone: (_____) _____

Email: _____

Personal Prayer Concerns:

_____
_____
_____
_____
_____
_____
_____

This form is for prayer requests that are personal to you and your journey in First Place 4 Health. Please complete this form and have it ready to turn in when you arrive at your group meeting.

First Place 4 Health
Prayer Partner

GROWING IN THE
FRUIT OF THE SPIRIT
Week
3

SCRIPTURE VERSE TO MEMORIZE FOR WEEK FOUR:

And without faith it is impossible to please God, because anyone who comes to him must believe that he exists and that he rewards those who earnestly seek him.

HEBREWS 11:6

Date: _____

Name: _____

Home Phone: (_____) _____

Work Phone: (_____) _____

Email: _____

Personal Prayer Concerns:

_____

_____

_____

_____

_____

_____

_____

This form is for prayer requests that are personal to you and your journey in First Place 4 Health. Please complete this form and have it ready to turn in when you arrive at your group meeting.

First Place 4 Health
Prayer Partner

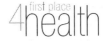

SCRIPTURE VERSE TO MEMORIZE FOR WEEK FIVE:

But the fruit of the Spirit is love, joy, peace, patience, kindness, goodness, faithfulness, gentleness and self-control. Against such things there is no law.

GALATIANS 5:22-23

Date: _____

Name: _____

Home Phone: (_____) _____

Work Phone: (_____) _____

Email: _____

Personal Prayer Concerns:

_____

_____

_____

_____

_____

_____

_____

This form is for prayer requests that are personal to you and your journey in First Place 4 Health. Please complete this form and have it ready to turn in when you arrive at your group meeting.

First Place 4 Health
Prayer Partner

4 first place health

SCRIPTURE VERSE TO MEMORIZE FOR WEEK SIX:
Do not grieve, for the joy of the LORD is your strength.
NEHEMIAH 8:10

Date: _____

Name: _____

Home Phone: (_____) _____

Work Phone: (_____) _____

Email: _____

Personal Prayer Concerns:

_____

_____

_____

_____

_____

_____

_____

This form is for prayer requests that are personal to you and your journey in First Place 4 Health. Please complete this form and have it ready to turn in when you arrive at your group meeting.

First Place 4 Health
Prayer Partner

GROWING IN THE
FRUIT OF THE SPIRIT
Week
6

SCRIPTURE VERSE TO MEMORIZE FOR WEEK SEVEN:

And the peace of God, which transcends all understanding,
will guard your hearts and your minds in Christ Jesus.

PHILIPPIANS 4:7

Date: _____

Name: _____

Home Phone: (_____) _____

Work Phone: (_____) _____

Email: _____

Personal Prayer Concerns:

_____

_____

_____

_____

_____

_____

_____

This form is for prayer requests that are personal to you and your journey in First Place 4 Health. Please complete this form and have it ready to turn in when you arrive at your group meeting.

First Place 4 Health
Prayer Partner

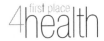

SCRIPTURE VERSE TO MEMORIZE FOR WEEK EIGHT:

*Let us not become weary in doing good, for at the proper time
we will reap a harvest if we do not give up.*

GALATIANS 6:9

Date: _____

Name: _____

Home Phone: (_____) _____

Work Phone: (_____) _____

Email: _____

Personal Prayer Concerns:

_____

_____

_____

_____

_____

_____

_____

This form is for prayer requests that are personal to you and your journey in First Place 4 Health. Please complete this form and have it ready to turn in when you arrive at your group meeting.

First Place 4 Health
Prayer Partner

4 first place
health

GROWING IN THE
FRUIT OF THE SPIRIT
Week
8

SCRIPTURE VERSE TO MEMORIZE FOR WEEK NINE:

Therefore, as God's chosen people, holy and dearly loved, clothe yourselves
with compassion, kindness, humility, gentleness and patience.

COLOSSIANS 3:12

Date: _____

Name: _____

Home Phone: (_____) _____

Work Phone: (_____) _____

Email: _____

Personal Prayer Concerns:

_____

_____

_____

_____

_____

_____

_____

This form is for prayer requests that are personal to you and your journey in First Place 4 Health. Please complete this form and have it ready to turn in when you arrive at your group meeting.

First Place 4 Health
Prayer Partner

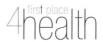

SCRIPTURE VERSE TO MEMORIZE FOR WEEK TEN:

*Take my yoke upon you and learn from me, for I am gentle and humble
in heart, and you will find rest for your souls.*

MATTHEW 11:29

Date: _____

Name: _____

Home Phone: (_____) _____

Work Phone: (_____) _____

Email: _____

Personal Prayer Concerns:

_____

_____

_____

_____

_____

_____

_____

This form is for prayer requests that are personal to you and your journey in First Place 4 Health. Please complete this
form and have it ready to turn in when you arrive at your group meeting.

First Place 4 Health
Prayer Partner

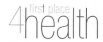

SCRIPTURE VERSE TO MEMORIZE FOR WEEK ELEVEN:

*So I say, live by the Spirit, and you will not gratify
the desires of the sinful nature.*

GALATIANS 5:16

Date: _____

Name: _____

Home Phone: _____

Work Phone: _____

Email: _____

Personal Prayer Concerns:

_____

_____

_____

_____

_____

_____

_____

This form is for prayer requests that are personal to you and your journey in First Place 4 Health. Please complete this form and have it ready to turn in when you arrive at your group meeting.

First Place 4 Health
Prayer Partner

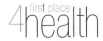

Date: _____

Name: _____

Home Phone: (_____) _____

Work Phone: (_____) _____

Email: _____

Personal Prayer Concerns:

_____

_____

_____

_____

_____

_____

_____

This form is for prayer requests that are personal to you and your journey in First Place 4 Health. Please complete this form and have it ready to turn in when you arrive at your group meeting.

Live It Tracker

Name: _____ Loss/gain: _____ lbs.

Date: _____ Week #: ____ Calorie Range: _____ My food goal for next week: _____

Activity Level: None, < 30 min/day, 30-60 min/day, 60+ min/day My activity goal for next week: _____

Group	Daily Calories							
	1300-1400	1500-1600	1700-1800	1900-2000	2100-2200	2300-2400	2500-2600	2700-2800
Fruits	1.5-2 c.	1.5-2 c.	1.5-2 c.	2-2.5 c.	2-2.5 c.	2.5-3.5 c.	3.5-4.5 c.	3.5-4.5 c.
Vegetables	1.5-2 c.	2-2.5 c.	2.5-3 c.	2.5-3 c.	3-3.5 c.	3.5-4.5 c.	4.5-5 c.	4.5-5 c.
Grains	5 oz-eq.	5-6 oz-eq.	6-7 oz-eq.	6-7 oz-eq.	7-8 oz-eq.	8-9 oz-eq.	9-10 oz-eq.	10-11 oz-eq.
Meat & Beans	4 oz-eq.	5 oz-eq.	5-5.5 oz-eq.	5.5-6.5 oz-eq.	6.5-7 oz-eq.	7-7.5 oz-eq.	7-7.5 oz-eq.	7.5-8 oz-eq.
Milk	2-3 c.	3 c.	3 c.	3 c.	3 c.	3 c.	3 c.	3 c.
Healthy Oils	4 tsp.	5 tsp.	5 tsp.	6 tsp.	6 tsp.	7 tsp.	8 tsp.	8 tsp.

Breakfast: _____ Lunch: _____

Dinner: _____ Snack: _____

Day/Date:

Group	Fruits	Vegetables	Grains	Meat & Beans	Milk	Oils
Goal Amount						
Estimate Your Total						
Increase ⬆ or Decrease? ⬇						

Physical Activity: _____ Spiritual Activity: _____

Steps/Miles/Minutes: _____

Breakfast: _____ Lunch: _____

Dinner: _____ Snack: _____

Day/Date:

Group	Fruits	Vegetables	Grains	Meat & Beans	Milk	Oils
Goal Amount						
Estimate Your Total						
Increase ⬆ or Decrease? ⬇						

Physical Activity: _____ Spiritual Activity: _____

Steps/Miles/Minutes: _____

Breakfast: _____ Lunch: _____

Dinner: _____ Snack: _____

Day/Date:

Group	Fruits	Vegetables	Grains	Meat & Beans	Milk	Oils
Goal Amount						
Estimate Your Total						
Increase ⬆ or Decrease? ⬇						

Physical Activity: _____ Spiritual Activity: _____

Steps/Miles/Minutes: _____

Day/Date: ___

Breakfast: _____ Lunch: _____

Dinner: _____ Snack: _____

Group	Fruits	Vegetables	Grains	Meat & Beans	Milk	Oils
Goal Amount						
Estimate Your Total						
Increase ⬆ or Decrease? ⬇						

Physical Activity: _____ Spiritual Activity: _____

Steps/Miles/Minutes: _____ _____

Day/Date: ___

Breakfast: _____ Lunch: _____

Dinner: _____ Snack: _____

Group	Fruits	Vegetables	Grains	Meat & Beans	Milk	Oils
Goal Amount						
Estimate Your Total						
Increase ⬆ or Decrease? ⬇						

Physical Activity: _____ Spiritual Activity: _____

Steps/Miles/Minutes: _____ _____

Day/Date: ___

Breakfast: _____ Lunch: _____

Dinner: _____ Snack: _____

Group	Fruits	Vegetables	Grains	Meat & Beans	Milk	Oils
Goal Amount						
Estimate Your Total						
Increase ⬆ or Decrease? ⬇						

Physical Activity: _____ Spiritual Activity: _____

Steps/Miles/Minutes: _____ _____

Day/Date: ___

Breakfast: _____ Lunch: _____

Dinner: _____ Snack: _____

Group	Fruits	Vegetables	Grains	Meat & Beans	Milk	Oils
Goal Amount						
Estimate Your Total						
Increase ⬆ or Decrease? ⬇						

Physical Activity: _____ Spiritual Activity: _____

Steps/Miles/Minutes: _____ _____

Live It Tracker

Name: _____ Loss/gain: _____ lbs.

Date: _____ Week #: _____ Calorie Range: _____ My food goal for next week: _____

Activity Level: None, < 30 min/day, 30-60 min/day, 60+ min/day My activity goal for next week: _____

Group	Daily Calories							
	1300-1400	1500-1600	1700-1800	1900-2000	2100-2200	2300-2400	2500-2600	2700-2800
Fruits	1.5-2 c.	1.5-2 c.	1.5-2 c.	2-2.5 c.	2-2.5 c.	2.5-3.5 c.	3.5-4.5 c.	3.5-4.5 c.
Vegetables	1.5-2 c.	2-2.5 c.	2.5-3 c.	2.5-3 c.	3-3.5 c.	3.5-4.5 c.	4.5-5 c.	4.5-5 c.
Grains	5 oz-eq.	5-6 oz-eq.	6-7 oz-eq.	6-7 oz-eq.	7-8 oz-eq.	8-9 oz-eq.	9-10 oz-eq.	10-11 oz-eq.
Meat & Beans	4 oz-eq.	5 oz-eq.	5-5.5 oz-eq.	5.5-6.5 oz-eq.	6.5-7 oz-eq.	7-7.5 oz-eq.	7-7.5 oz-eq.	7.5-8 oz-eq.
Milk	2-3 c.	3 c.	3 c.	3 c.	3 c.	3 c.	3 c.	3 c.
Healthy Oils	4 tsp.	5 tsp.	5 tsp.	6 tsp.	6 tsp.	7 tsp.	8 tsp.	8 tsp.

Day/Date:

Breakfast: _____ Lunch: _____

Dinner: _____ Snack: _____

Group	Fruits	Vegetables	Grains	Meat & Beans	Milk	Oils
Goal Amount						
Estimate Your Total						
Increase ⇧ or Decrease? ⇩						

Physical Activity: _____ Spiritual Activity: _____

Steps/Miles/Minutes: _____

Day/Date:

Breakfast: _____ Lunch: _____

Dinner: _____ Snack: _____

Group	Fruits	Vegetables	Grains	Meat & Beans	Milk	Oils
Goal Amount						
Estimate Your Total						
Increase ⇧ or Decrease? ⇩						

Physical Activity: _____ Spiritual Activity: _____

Steps/Miles/Minutes: _____

Day/Date:

Breakfast: _____ Lunch: _____

Dinner: _____ Snack: _____

Group	Fruits	Vegetables	Grains	Meat & Beans	Milk	Oils
Goal Amount						
Estimate Your Total						
Increase ⇧ or Decrease? ⇩						

Physical Activity: _____ Spiritual Activity: _____

Steps/Miles/Minutes: _____

Breakfast: _____ **Lunch:** _____

Dinner: _____ **Snack:** _____

Group	Fruits	Vegetables	Grains	Meat & Beans	Milk	Oils
Goal Amount						
Estimate Your Total						
Increase ⇧ or Decrease? ⇩						

Physical Activity: _____ **Spiritual Activity:** _____

Steps/Miles/Minutes: _____

Breakfast: _____ **Lunch:** _____

Dinner: _____ **Snack:** _____

Group	Fruits	Vegetables	Grains	Meat & Beans	Milk	Oils
Goal Amount						
Estimate Your Total						
Increase ⇧ or Decrease? ⇩						

Physical Activity: _____ **Spiritual Activity:** _____

Steps/Miles/Minutes: _____

Breakfast: _____ **Lunch:** _____

Dinner: _____ **Snack:** _____

Group	Fruits	Vegetables	Grains	Meat & Beans	Milk	Oils
Goal Amount						
Estimate Your Total						
Increase ⇧ or Decrease? ⇩						

Physical Activity: _____ **Spiritual Activity:** _____

Steps/Miles/Minutes: _____

Breakfast: _____ **Lunch:** _____

Dinner: _____ **Snack:** _____

Group	Fruits	Vegetables	Grains	Meat & Beans	Milk	Oils
Goal Amount						
Estimate Your Total						
Increase ⇧ or Decrease? ⇩						

Physical Activity: _____ **Spiritual Activity:** _____

Steps/Miles/Minutes: _____

Day/Date: _____

Live It Tracker

Name: _____ Loss/gain: _____ lbs.

Date: _____ Week #: _____ Calorie Range: _____ My food goal for next week: _____

Activity Level: None, < 30 min/day, 30-60 min/day, 60+ min/day My activity goal for next week: _____

Group	Daily Calories							
	1300-1400	1500-1600	1700-1800	1900-2000	2100-2200	2300-2400	2500-2600	2700-2800
Fruits	1.5-2 c.	1.5-2 c.	1.5-2 c.	2-2.5 c.	2-2.5 c.	2.5-3.5 c.	3.5-4.5 c.	3.5-4.5 c.
Vegetables	1.5-2 c.	2-2.5 c.	2.5-3 c.	2.5-3 c.	3-3.5 c.	3.5-4.5 c.	4.5-5 c.	4.5-5 c.
Grains	5 oz-eq.	5-6 oz-eq.	6-7 oz-eq.	6-7 oz-eq.	7-8 oz-eq.	8-9 oz-eq.	9-10 oz-eq.	10-11 oz-eq.
Meat & Beans	4 oz-eq.	5 oz-eq.	5-5.5 oz-eq.	5.5-6.5 oz-eq.	6.5-7 oz-eq.	7-7.5 oz-eq.	7-7.5 oz-eq.	7.5-8 oz-eq.
Milk	2-3 c.	3 c.	3 c.	3 c.	3 c.	3 c.	3 c.	3 c.
Healthy Oils	4 tsp.	5 tsp.	5 tsp.	6 tsp.	6 tsp.	7 tsp.	8 tsp.	8 tsp.

Breakfast: _____ Lunch: _____

Dinner: _____ Snack: _____

Day/Date:

Group	Fruits	Vegetables	Grains	Meat & Beans	Milk	Oils
Goal Amount						
Estimate Your Total						
Increase ⇧ or Decrease? ⇩						

Physical Activity: _____ Spiritual Activity: _____

Steps/Miles/Minutes: _____

Breakfast: _____ Lunch: _____

Dinner: _____ Snack: _____

Day/Date:

Group	Fruits	Vegetables	Grains	Meat & Beans	Milk	Oils
Goal Amount						
Estimate Your Total						
Increase ⇧ or Decrease? ⇩						

Physical Activity: _____ Spiritual Activity: _____

Steps/Miles/Minutes: _____

Breakfast: _____ Lunch: _____

Dinner: _____ Snack: _____

Day/Date:

Group	Fruits	Vegetables	Grains	Meat & Beans	Milk	Oils
Goal Amount						
Estimate Your Total						
Increase ⇧ or Decrease? ⇩						

Physical Activity: _____ Spiritual Activity: _____

Steps/Miles/Minutes: _____

Breakfast: _____   Lunch: _____

Dinner: _____   Snack: _____
_____   _____

Group	Fruits	Vegetables	Grains	Meat & Beans	Milk	Oils
Goal Amount						
Estimate Your Total						
Increase ⬆ or Decrease? ⬇						

Physical Activity: _____   Spiritual Activity: _____

Steps/Miles/Minutes: _____   _____

Day/Date:

Breakfast: _____   Lunch: _____

Dinner: _____   Snack: _____
_____   _____

Group	Fruits	Vegetables	Grains	Meat & Beans	Milk	Oils
Goal Amount						
Estimate Your Total						
Increase ⬆ or Decrease? ⬇						

Physical Activity: _____   Spiritual Activity: _____

Steps/Miles/Minutes: _____   _____

Day/Date:

Breakfast: _____   Lunch: _____

Dinner: _____   Snack: _____
_____   _____

Group	Fruits	Vegetables	Grains	Meat & Beans	Milk	Oils
Goal Amount						
Estimate Your Total						
Increase ⬆ or Decrease? ⬇						

Physical Activity: _____   Spiritual Activity: _____

Steps/Miles/Minutes: _____   _____

Day/Date:

Breakfast: _____   Lunch: _____

Dinner: _____   Snack: _____
_____   _____

Group	Fruits	Vegetables	Grains	Meat & Beans	Milk	Oils
Goal Amount						
Estimate Your Total						
Increase ⬆ or Decrease? ⬇						

Physical Activity: _____   Spiritual Activity: _____

Steps/Miles/Minutes: _____   _____

Day/Date:

Live It Tracker

Name: _____ Loss/gain: _____ lbs.

Date: _____ Week #: ____ Calorie Range: _____ My food goal for next week: _____

Activity Level: None, < 30 min/day, 30-60 min/day, 60+ min/day My activity goal for next week: _____

Group	Daily Calories							
	1300-1400	1500-1600	1700-1800	1900-2000	2100-2200	2300-2400	2500-2600	2700-2800
Fruits	1.5-2 c.	1.5-2 c.	1.5-2 c.	2-2.5 c.	2-2.5 c.	2.5-3.5 c.	3.5-4.5 c.	3.5-4.5 c.
Vegetables	1.5-2 c.	2-2.5 c.	2.5-3 c.	2.5-3 c.	3-3.5 c.	3.5-4.5 c.	4.5-5 c.	4.5-5 c.
Grains	5 oz-eq.	5-6 oz-eq.	6-7 oz-eq.	6-7 oz-eq.	7-8 oz-eq.	8-9 oz-eq.	9-10 oz-eq.	10-11 oz-eq.
Meat & Beans	4 oz-eq.	5 oz-eq.	5-5.5 oz-eq.	5.5-6.5 oz-eq.	6.5-7 oz-eq.	7-7.5 oz-eq.	7-7.5 oz-eq.	7.5-8 oz-eq.
Milk	2-3 c.	3 c.	3 c.	3 c.	3 c.	3 c.	3 c.	3 c.
Healthy Oils	4 tsp.	5 tsp.	5 tsp.	6 tsp.	6 tsp.	7 tsp.	8 tsp.	8 tsp.

Day/Date: _____

Breakfast: _____ Lunch: _____

Dinner: _____ Snack: _____

Group	Fruits	Vegetables	Grains	Meat & Beans	Milk	Oils
Goal Amount						
Estimate Your Total						
Increase ⇧ or Decrease? ⇩						

Physical Activity: _____ Spiritual Activity: _____

Steps/Miles/Minutes: _____

Day/Date: _____

Breakfast: _____ Lunch: _____

Dinner: _____ Snack: _____

Group	Fruits	Vegetables	Grains	Meat & Beans	Milk	Oils
Goal Amount						
Estimate Your Total						
Increase ⇧ or Decrease? ⇩						

Physical Activity: _____ Spiritual Activity: _____

Steps/Miles/Minutes: _____

Day/Date: _____

Breakfast: _____ Lunch: _____

Dinner: _____ Snack: _____

Group	Fruits	Vegetables	Grains	Meat & Beans	Milk	Oils
Goal Amount						
Estimate Your Total						
Increase ⇧ or Decrease? ⇩						

Physical Activity: _____ Spiritual Activity: _____

Steps/Miles/Minutes: _____

Day/Date: ___

Breakfast: _____ Lunch: _____

Dinner: _____ Snack: _____

Group	Fruits	Vegetables	Grains	Meat & Beans	Milk	Oils
Goal Amount						
Estimate Your Total						
Increase ⇧ or Decrease? ⇩						

Physical Activity: _____ Spiritual Activity: _____

Steps/Miles/Minutes: _____ _____

Day/Date: ___

Breakfast: _____ Lunch: _____

Dinner: _____ Snack: _____

Group	Fruits	Vegetables	Grains	Meat & Beans	Milk	Oils
Goal Amount						
Estimate Your Total						
Increase ⇧ or Decrease? ⇩						

Physical Activity: _____ Spiritual Activity: _____

Steps/Miles/Minutes: _____ _____

Day/Date: ___

Breakfast: _____ Lunch: _____

Dinner: _____ Snack: _____

Group	Fruits	Vegetables	Grains	Meat & Beans	Milk	Oils
Goal Amount						
Estimate Your Total						
Increase ⇧ or Decrease? ⇩						

Physical Activity: _____ Spiritual Activity: _____

Steps/Miles/Minutes: _____ _____

Day/Date: ___

Breakfast: _____ Lunch: _____

Dinner: _____ Snack: _____

Group	Fruits	Vegetables	Grains	Meat & Beans	Milk	Oils
Goal Amount						
Estimate Your Total						
Increase ⇧ or Decrease? ⇩						

Physical Activity: _____ Spiritual Activity: _____

Steps/Miles/Minutes: _____ _____

Live It Tracker

Name: _____ Loss/gain: _____ lbs.

Date: _____ Week #: _____ Calorie Range: _____ My food goal for next week: _____

Activity Level: None, < 30 min/day, 30-60 min/day, 60+ min/day My activity goal for next week: _____

Group	Daily Calories							
	1300-1400	1500-1600	1700-1800	1900-2000	2100-2200	2300-2400	2500-2600	2700-2800
Fruits	1.5-2 c.	1.5-2 c.	1.5-2 c.	2-2.5 c.	2-2.5 c.	2.5-3.5 c.	3.5-4.5 c.	3.5-4.5 c.
Vegetables	1.5-2 c.	2-2.5 c.	2.5-3 c.	2.5-3 c.	3-3.5 c.	3.5-4.5 c.	4.5-5 c.	4.5-5 c.
Grains	5 oz-eq.	5-6 oz-eq.	6-7 oz-eq.	6-7 oz-eq.	7-8 oz-eq.	8-9 oz-eq.	9-10 oz-eq.	10-11 oz-eq.
Meat & Beans	4 oz-eq.	5 oz-eq.	5-5.5 oz-eq.	5.5-6.5 oz-eq.	6.5-7 oz-eq.	7-7.5 oz-eq.	7-7.5 oz-eq.	7.5-8 oz-eq.
Milk	2-3 c.	3 c.	3 c.	3 c.	3 c.	3 c.	3 c.	3 c.
Healthy Oils	4 tsp.	5 tsp.	5 tsp.	6 tsp.	6 tsp.	7 tsp.	8 tsp.	8 tsp.

Day/Date:

Breakfast: _____ Lunch: _____

Dinner: _____ Snack: _____

Group	Fruits	Vegetables	Grains	Meat & Beans	Milk	Oils
Goal Amount						
Estimate Your Total						
Increase ⇧ or Decrease? ⇩						

Physical Activity: _____ Spiritual Activity: _____

Steps/Miles/Minutes: _____

Day/Date:

Breakfast: _____ Lunch: _____

Dinner: _____ Snack: _____

Group	Fruits	Vegetables	Grains	Meat & Beans	Milk	Oils
Goal Amount						
Estimate Your Total						
Increase ⇧ or Decrease? ⇩						

Physical Activity: _____ Spiritual Activity: _____

Steps/Miles/Minutes: _____

Day/Date:

Breakfast: _____ Lunch: _____

Dinner: _____ Snack: _____

Group	Fruits	Vegetables	Grains	Meat & Beans	Milk	Oils
Goal Amount						
Estimate Your Total						
Increase ⇧ or Decrease? ⇩						

Physical Activity: _____ Spiritual Activity: _____

Steps/Miles/Minutes: _____

Day/Date: _____

Breakfast: _____   Lunch: _____

Dinner: _____   Snack: _____

Group	Fruits	Vegetables	Grains	Meat & Beans	Milk	Oils
Goal Amount						
Estimate Your Total						
Increase ⇧ or Decrease? ⇩						

Physical Activity: _____   Spiritual Activity: _____

Steps/Miles/Minutes: _____   _____

Day/Date: _____

Breakfast: _____   Lunch: _____

Dinner: _____   Snack: _____

Group	Fruits	Vegetables	Grains	Meat & Beans	Milk	Oils
Goal Amount						
Estimate Your Total						
Increase ⇧ or Decrease? ⇩						

Physical Activity: _____   Spiritual Activity: _____

Steps/Miles/Minutes: _____   _____

Day/Date: _____

Breakfast: _____   Lunch: _____

Dinner: _____   Snack: _____

Group	Fruits	Vegetables	Grains	Meat & Beans	Milk	Oils
Goal Amount						
Estimate Your Total						
Increase ⇧ or Decrease? ⇩						

Physical Activity: _____   Spiritual Activity: _____

Steps/Miles/Minutes: _____   _____

Day/Date: _____

Breakfast: _____   Lunch: _____

Dinner: _____   Snack: _____

Group	Fruits	Vegetables	Grains	Meat & Beans	Milk	Oils
Goal Amount						
Estimate Your Total						
Increase ⇧ or Decrease? ⇩						

Physical Activity: _____   Spiritual Activity: _____

Steps/Miles/Minutes: _____   _____

Live It Tracker

Name: _____ Loss/gain: _____ lbs.

Date: _____ Week #: _____ Calorie Range: _____ My food goal for next week: _____

Activity Level: None, < 30 min/day, 30-60 min/day, 60+ min/day My activity goal for next week: _____

Group	Daily Calories							
	1300-1400	1500-1600	1700-1800	1900-2000	2100-2200	2300-2400	2500-2600	2700-2800
Fruits	1.5-2 c.	1.5-2 c.	1.5-2 c.	2-2.5 c.	2-2.5 c.	2.5-3.5 c.	3.5-4.5 c.	3.5-4.5 c.
Vegetables	1.5-2 c.	2-2.5 c.	2.5-3 c.	2.5-3 c.	3-3.5 c.	3.5-4.5 c.	4.5-5 c.	4.5-5 c.
Grains	5 oz-eq.	5-6 oz-eq.	6-7 oz-eq.	6-7 oz-eq.	7-8 oz-eq.	8-9 oz-eq.	9-10 oz-eq.	10-11 oz-eq.
Meat & Beans	4 oz-eq.	5 oz-eq.	5-5.5 oz-eq.	5.5-6.5 oz-eq.	6.5-7 oz-eq.	7-7.5 oz-eq.	7-7.5 oz-eq.	7.5-8 oz-eq.
Milk	2-3 c.	3 c.	3 c.	3 c.	3 c.	3 c.	3 c.	3 c.
Healthy Oils	4 tsp.	5 tsp.	5 tsp.	6 tsp.	6 tsp.	7 tsp.	8 tsp.	8 tsp.

Day/Date: _____

Breakfast: _____ Lunch: _____

Dinner: _____ Snack: _____

Group	Fruits	Vegetables	Grains	Meat & Beans	Milk	Oils
Goal Amount						
Estimate Your Total						
Increase ⇧ or Decrease? ⇩						

Physical Activity: _____ Spiritual Activity: _____

Steps/Miles/Minutes: _____

Day/Date: _____

Breakfast: _____ Lunch: _____

Dinner: _____ Snack: _____

Group	Fruits	Vegetables	Grains	Meat & Beans	Milk	Oils
Goal Amount						
Estimate Your Total						
Increase ⇧ or Decrease? ⇩						

Physical Activity: _____ Spiritual Activity: _____

Steps/Miles/Minutes: _____

Day/Date: _____

Breakfast: _____ Lunch: _____

Dinner: _____ Snack: _____

Group	Fruits	Vegetables	Grains	Meat & Beans	Milk	Oils
Goal Amount						
Estimate Your Total						
Increase ⇧ or Decrease? ⇩						

Physical Activity: _____ Spiritual Activity: _____

Steps/Miles/Minutes: _____

Day/Date:

Breakfast: _____ Lunch: _____

Dinner: _____ Snack: _____

Group	Fruits	Vegetables	Grains	Meat & Beans	Milk	Oils
Goal Amount						
Estimate Your Total						
Increase ⬆ or Decrease? ⬇						

Physical Activity: _____ Spiritual Activity: _____

Steps/Miles/Minutes: _____

Day/Date:

Breakfast: _____ Lunch: _____

Dinner: _____ Snack: _____

Group	Fruits	Vegetables	Grains	Meat & Beans	Milk	Oils
Goal Amount						
Estimate Your Total						
Increase ⬆ or Decrease? ⬇						

Physical Activity: _____ Spiritual Activity: _____

Steps/Miles/Minutes: _____

Day/Date:

Breakfast: _____ Lunch: _____

Dinner: _____ Snack: _____

Group	Fruits	Vegetables	Grains	Meat & Beans	Milk	Oils
Goal Amount						
Estimate Your Total						
Increase ⬆ or Decrease? ⬇						

Physical Activity: _____ Spiritual Activity: _____

Steps/Miles/Minutes: _____

Day/Date:

Breakfast: _____ Lunch: _____

Dinner: _____ Snack: _____

Group	Fruits	Vegetables	Grains	Meat & Beans	Milk	Oils
Goal Amount						
Estimate Your Total						
Increase ⬆ or Decrease? ⬇						

Physical Activity: _____ Spiritual Activity: _____

Steps/Miles/Minutes: _____

Live It Tracker

Name: _____   Loss/gain: _____ lbs.

Date: _____ Week #: _____ Calorie Range: _____ My food goal for next week: _____

Activity Level: None, < 30 min/day, 30-60 min/day, 60+ min/day   My activity goal for next week: _____

Group	Daily Calories							
	1300-1400	1500-1600	1700-1800	1900-2000	2100-2200	2300-2400	2500-2600	2700-2800
Fruits	1.5-2 c.	1.5-2 c.	1.5-2 c.	2-2.5 c.	2-2.5 c.	2.5-3.5 c.	3.5-4.5 c.	3.5-4.5 c.
Vegetables	1.5-2 c.	2-2.5 c.	2.5-3 c.	2.5-3 c.	3-3.5 c.	3.5-4.5 c.	4.5-5 c.	4.5-5 c.
Grains	5 oz-eq.	5-6 oz-eq.	6-7 oz-eq.	6-7 oz-eq.	7-8 oz-eq.	8-9 oz-eq.	9-10 oz-eq.	10-11 oz-eq.
Meat & Beans	4 oz-eq.	5 oz-eq.	5-5.5 oz-eq.	5.5-6.5 oz-eq.	6.5-7 oz-eq.	7-7.5 oz-eq.	7-7.5 oz-eq.	7.5-8 oz-eq.
Milk	2-3 c.	3 c.	3 c.	3 c.	3 c.	3 c.	3 c.	3 c.
Healthy Oils	4 tsp.	5 tsp.	5 tsp.	6 tsp.	6 tsp.	7 tsp.	8 tsp.	8 tsp.

Day/Date:

Breakfast: _____   Lunch: _____

Dinner: _____   Snack: _____

Group	Fruits	Vegetables	Grains	Meat & Beans	Milk	Oils
Goal Amount						
Estimate Your Total						
Increase ⇧ or Decrease? ⇩						

Physical Activity: _____   Spiritual Activity: _____

Steps/Miles/Minutes: _____

Day/Date:

Breakfast: _____   Lunch: _____

Dinner: _____   Snack: _____

Group	Fruits	Vegetables	Grains	Meat & Beans	Milk	Oils
Goal Amount						
Estimate Your Total						
Increase ⇧ or Decrease? ⇩						

Physical Activity: _____   Spiritual Activity: _____

Steps/Miles/Minutes: _____

Day/Date:

Breakfast: _____   Lunch: _____

Dinner: _____   Snack: _____

Group	Fruits	Vegetables	Grains	Meat & Beans	Milk	Oils
Goal Amount						
Estimate Your Total						
Increase ⇧ or Decrease? ⇩						

Physical Activity: _____   Spiritual Activity: _____

Steps/Miles/Minutes: _____

Day/Date:

Breakfast: _____ Lunch: _____

Dinner: _____ Snack: _____

Group	Fruits	Vegetables	Grains	Meat & Beans	Milk	Oils
Goal Amount						
Estimate Your Total						
Increase ⇧ or Decrease? ⇩						

Physical Activity: _____ Spiritual Activity: _____

Steps/Miles/Minutes: _____ _____

Day/Date:

Breakfast: _____ Lunch: _____

Dinner: _____ Snack: _____

Group	Fruits	Vegetables	Grains	Meat & Beans	Milk	Oils
Goal Amount						
Estimate Your Total						
Increase ⇧ or Decrease? ⇩						

Physical Activity: _____ Spiritual Activity: _____

Steps/Miles/Minutes: _____ _____

Day/Date:

Breakfast: _____ Lunch: _____

Dinner: _____ Snack: _____

Group	Fruits	Vegetables	Grains	Meat & Beans	Milk	Oils
Goal Amount						
Estimate Your Total						
Increase ⇧ or Decrease? ⇩						

Physical Activity: _____ Spiritual Activity: _____

Steps/Miles/Minutes: _____ _____

Day/Date:

Breakfast: _____ Lunch: _____

Dinner: _____ Snack: _____

Group	Fruits	Vegetables	Grains	Meat & Beans	Milk	Oils
Goal Amount						
Estimate Your Total						
Increase ⇧ or Decrease? ⇩						

Physical Activity: _____ Spiritual Activity: _____

Steps/Miles/Minutes: _____ _____

Live It Tracker

Name: _____ Loss/gain: _____ lbs.

Date: _____ Week #: ____ Calorie Range: _____ My food goal for next week: _____

Activity Level: None, < 30 min/day, 30-60 min/day, 60+ min/day My activity goal for next week: _____

Group	Daily Calories							
	1300-1400	1500-1600	1700-1800	1900-2000	2100-2200	2300-2400	2500-2600	2700-2800
Fruits	1.5-2 c.	1.5-2 c.	1.5-2 c.	2-2.5 c.	2-2.5 c.	2.5-3.5 c.	3.5-4.5 c.	3.5-4.5 c.
Vegetables	1.5-2 c.	2-2.5 c.	2.5-3 c.	2.5-3 c.	3-3.5 c.	3.5-4.5 c.	4.5-5 c.	4.5-5 c.
Grains	5 oz-eq.	5-6 oz-eq.	6-7 oz-eq.	6-7 oz-eq.	7-8 oz-eq.	8-9 oz-eq.	9-10 oz-eq.	10-11 oz-eq.
Meat & Beans	4 oz-eq.	5 oz-eq.	5-5.5 oz-eq.	5.5-6.5 oz-eq.	6.5-7 oz-eq.	7-7.5 oz-eq.	7-7.5 oz-eq.	7.5-8 oz-eq.
Milk	2-3 c.	3 c.	3 c.	3 c.	3 c.	3 c.	3 c.	3 c.
Healthy Oils	4 tsp.	5 tsp.	5 tsp.	6 tsp.	6 tsp.	7 tsp.	8 tsp.	8 tsp.

Day/Date:

Breakfast: _____ Lunch: _____

Dinner: _____ Snack: _____

Group	Fruits	Vegetables	Grains	Meat & Beans	Milk	Oils
Goal Amount						
Estimate Your Total						
Increase ⇧ or Decrease? ⇩						

Physical Activity: _____ Spiritual Activity: _____

Steps/Miles/Minutes: _____

Day/Date:

Breakfast: _____ Lunch: _____

Dinner: _____ Snack: _____

Group	Fruits	Vegetables	Grains	Meat & Beans	Milk	Oils
Goal Amount						
Estimate Your Total						
Increase ⇧ or Decrease? ⇩						

Physical Activity: _____ Spiritual Activity: _____

Steps/Miles/Minutes: _____

Day/Date:

Breakfast: _____ Lunch: _____

Dinner: _____ Snack: _____

Group	Fruits	Vegetables	Grains	Meat & Beans	Milk	Oils
Goal Amount						
Estimate Your Total						
Increase ⇧ or Decrease? ⇩						

Physical Activity: _____ Spiritual Activity: _____

Steps/Miles/Minutes: _____

Day/Date: _____

Breakfast: _____   Lunch: _____

Dinner: _____   Snack: _____

Group	Fruits	Vegetables	Grains	Meat & Beans	Milk	Oils
Goal Amount						
Estimate Your Total						
Increase ⇧ or Decrease? ⇩						

Physical Activity: _____   Spiritual Activity: _____

Steps/Miles/Minutes: _____   _____

Day/Date: _____

Breakfast: _____   Lunch: _____

Dinner: _____   Snack: _____

Group	Fruits	Vegetables	Grains	Meat & Beans	Milk	Oils
Goal Amount						
Estimate Your Total						
Increase ⇧ or Decrease? ⇩						

Physical Activity: _____   Spiritual Activity: _____

Steps/Miles/Minutes: _____   _____

Day/Date: _____

Breakfast: _____   Lunch: _____

Dinner: _____   Snack: _____

Group	Fruits	Vegetables	Grains	Meat & Beans	Milk	Oils
Goal Amount						
Estimate Your Total						
Increase ⇧ or Decrease? ⇩						

Physical Activity: _____   Spiritual Activity: _____

Steps/Miles/Minutes: _____   _____

Day/Date: _____

Breakfast: _____   Lunch: _____

Dinner: _____   Snack: _____

Group	Fruits	Vegetables	Grains	Meat & Beans	Milk	Oils
Goal Amount						
Estimate Your Total						
Increase ⇧ or Decrease? ⇩						

Physical Activity: _____   Spiritual Activity: _____

Steps/Miles/Minutes: _____   _____

Live It Tracker

Name: _____ Loss/gain: _____ lbs.

Date: _____ Week #: _____ Calorie Range: _____ My food goal for next week: _____

Activity Level: None, < 30 min/day, 30-60 min/day, 60+ min/day My activity goal for next week: _____

Group	Daily Calories							
	1300-1400	1500-1600	1700-1800	1900-2000	2100-2200	2300-2400	2500-2600	2700-2800
Fruits	1.5-2 c.	1.5-2 c.	1.5-2 c.	2-2.5 c.	2-2.5 c.	2.5-3.5 c.	3.5-4.5 c.	3.5-4.5 c.
Vegetables	1.5-2 c.	2-2.5 c.	2.5-3 c.	2.5-3 c.	3-3.5 c.	3.5-4.5 c.	4.5-5 c.	4.5-5 c.
Grains	5 oz-eq.	5-6 oz-eq.	6-7 oz-eq.	6-7 oz-eq.	7-8 oz-eq.	8-9 oz-eq.	9-10 oz-eq.	10-11 oz-eq.
Meat & Beans	4 oz-eq.	5 oz-eq.	5-5.5 oz-eq.	5.5-6.5 oz-eq.	6.5-7 oz-eq.	7-7.5 oz-eq.	7-7.5 oz-eq.	7.5-8 oz-eq.
Milk	2-3 c.	3 c.	3 c.	3 c.	3 c.	3 c.	3 c.	3 c.
Healthy Oils	4 tsp.	5 tsp.	5 tsp.	6 tsp.	6 tsp.	7 tsp.	8 tsp.	8 tsp.

Day/Date: _____

Breakfast: _____ Lunch: _____

Dinner: _____ Snack: _____

Group	Fruits	Vegetables	Grains	Meat & Beans	Milk	Oils
Goal Amount						
Estimate Your Total						
Increase ⇧ or Decrease? ⇩						

Physical Activity: _____ Spiritual Activity: _____

Steps/Miles/Minutes: _____

Day/Date: _____

Breakfast: _____ Lunch: _____

Dinner: _____ Snack: _____

Group	Fruits	Vegetables	Grains	Meat & Beans	Milk	Oils
Goal Amount						
Estimate Your Total						
Increase ⇧ or Decrease? ⇩						

Physical Activity: _____ Spiritual Activity: _____

Steps/Miles/Minutes: _____

Day/Date: _____

Breakfast: _____ Lunch: _____

Dinner: _____ Snack: _____

Group	Fruits	Vegetables	Grains	Meat & Beans	Milk	Oils
Goal Amount						
Estimate Your Total						
Increase ⇧ or Decrease? ⇩						

Physical Activity: _____ Spiritual Activity: _____

Steps/Miles/Minutes: _____

Day/Date:

Breakfast: _____ Lunch: _____

Dinner: _____ Snack: _____

Group	Fruits	Vegetables	Grains	Meat & Beans	Milk	Oils
Goal Amount						
Estimate Your Total						
Increase ⇧ or Decrease? ⇩						

Physical Activity: _____ Spiritual Activity: _____

Steps/Miles/Minutes: _____ _____

Day/Date:

Breakfast: _____ Lunch: _____

Dinner: _____ Snack: _____

Group	Fruits	Vegetables	Grains	Meat & Beans	Milk	Oils
Goal Amount						
Estimate Your Total						
Increase ⇧ or Decrease? ⇩						

Physical Activity: _____ Spiritual Activity: _____

Steps/Miles/Minutes: _____ _____

Day/Date:

Breakfast: _____ Lunch: _____

Dinner: _____ Snack: _____

Group	Fruits	Vegetables	Grains	Meat & Beans	Milk	Oils
Goal Amount						
Estimate Your Total						
Increase ⇧ or Decrease? ⇩						

Physical Activity: _____ Spiritual Activity: _____

Steps/Miles/Minutes: _____ _____

Day/Date:

Breakfast: _____ Lunch: _____

Dinner: _____ Snack: _____

Group	Fruits	Vegetables	Grains	Meat & Beans	Milk	Oils
Goal Amount						
Estimate Your Total						
Increase ⇧ or Decrease? ⇩						

Physical Activity: _____ Spiritual Activity: _____

Steps/Miles/Minutes: _____ _____

Live It Tracker

Name: _____ Loss/gain: _____ lbs.

Date: _____ Week #: _____ Calorie Range: _____ My food goal for next week: _____

Activity Level: None, < 30 min/day, 30-60 min/day, 60+ min/day My activity goal for next week: _____

Group	Daily Calories							
	1300-1400	1500-1600	1700-1800	1900-2000	2100-2200	2300-2400	2500-2600	2700-2800
Fruits	1.5-2 c.	1.5-2 c.	1.5-2 c.	2-2.5 c.	2-2.5 c.	2.5-3.5 c.	3.5-4.5 c.	3.5-4.5 c.
Vegetables	1.5-2 c.	2-2.5 c.	2.5-3 c.	2.5-3 c.	3-3.5 c.	3.5-4.5 c.	4.5-5 c.	4.5-5 c.
Grains	5 oz-eq.	5-6 oz-eq.	6-7 oz-eq.	6-7 oz-eq.	7-8 oz-eq.	8-9 oz-eq.	9-10 oz-eq.	10-11 oz-eq.
Meat & Beans	4 oz-eq.	5 oz-eq.	5-5.5 oz-eq.	5.5-6.5 oz-eq.	6.5-7 oz-eq.	7-7.5 oz-eq.	7-7.5 oz-eq.	7.5-8 oz-eq.
Milk	2-3 c.	3 c.	3 c.	3 c.	3 c.	3 c.	3 c.	3 c.
Healthy Oils	4 tsp.	5 tsp.	5 tsp.	6 tsp.	6 tsp.	7 tsp.	8 tsp.	8 tsp.

Day/Date:

Breakfast: _____ Lunch: _____

Dinner: _____ Snack: _____

Group	Fruits	Vegetables	Grains	Meat & Beans	Milk	Oils
Goal Amount						
Estimate Your Total						
Increase ⇧ or Decrease? ⇩						

Physical Activity: _____ Spiritual Activity: _____

Steps/Miles/Minutes: _____

Day/Date:

Breakfast: _____ Lunch: _____

Dinner: _____ Snack: _____

Group	Fruits	Vegetables	Grains	Meat & Beans	Milk	Oils
Goal Amount						
Estimate Your Total						
Increase ⇧ or Decrease? ⇩						

Physical Activity: _____ Spiritual Activity: _____

Steps/Miles/Minutes: _____

Day/Date:

Breakfast: _____ Lunch: _____

Dinner: _____ Snack: _____

Group	Fruits	Vegetables	Grains	Meat & Beans	Milk	Oils
Goal Amount						
Estimate Your Total						
Increase ⇧ or Decrease? ⇩						

Physical Activity: _____ Spiritual Activity: _____

Steps/Miles/Minutes: _____

Day/Date: ___

Breakfast: _____ Lunch: _____

Dinner: _____ Snack: _____

Group	Fruits	Vegetables	Grains	Meat & Beans	Milk	Oils
Goal Amount						
Estimate Your Total						
Increase ⬆ or Decrease? ⬇						

Physical Activity: _____ Spiritual Activity: _____

Steps/Miles/Minutes: _____ _____

Day/Date: ___

Breakfast: _____ Lunch: _____

Dinner: _____ Snack: _____

Group	Fruits	Vegetables	Grains	Meat & Beans	Milk	Oils
Goal Amount						
Estimate Your Total						
Increase ⬆ or Decrease? ⬇						

Physical Activity: _____ Spiritual Activity: _____

Steps/Miles/Minutes: _____ _____

Day/Date: ___

Breakfast: _____ Lunch: _____

Dinner: _____ Snack: _____

Group	Fruits	Vegetables	Grains	Meat & Beans	Milk	Oils
Goal Amount						
Estimate Your Total						
Increase ⬆ or Decrease? ⬇						

Physical Activity: _____ Spiritual Activity: _____

Steps/Miles/Minutes: _____ _____

Day/Date: ___

Breakfast: _____ Lunch: _____

Dinner: _____ Snack: _____

Group	Fruits	Vegetables	Grains	Meat & Beans	Milk	Oils
Goal Amount						
Estimate Your Total						
Increase ⬆ or Decrease? ⬇						

Physical Activity: _____ Spiritual Activity: _____

Steps/Miles/Minutes: _____ _____

Live It Tracker

Name: _____ Loss/gain: _____ lbs.

Date: _____ Week #: _____ Calorie Range: _____ My food goal for next week: _____

Activity Level: None, < 30 min/day, 30-60 min/day, 60+ min/day My activity goal for next week: _____

Group	Daily Calories							
	1300-1400	1500-1600	1700-1800	1900-2000	2100-2200	2300-2400	2500-2600	2700-2800
Fruits	1.5-2 c.	1.5-2 c.	1.5-2 c.	2-2.5 c.	2-2.5 c.	2.5-3.5 c.	3.5-4.5 c.	3.5-4.5 c.
Vegetables	1.5-2 c.	2-2.5 c.	2.5-3 c.	2.5-3 c.	3-3.5 c.	3.5-4.5 c.	4.5-5 c.	4.5-5 c.
Grains	5 oz-eq.	5-6 oz-eq.	6-7 oz-eq.	6-7 oz-eq.	7-8 oz-eq.	8-9 oz-eq.	9-10 oz-eq.	10-11 oz-eq.
Meat & Beans	4 oz-eq.	5 oz-eq.	5-5.5 oz-eq.	5.5-6.5 oz-eq.	6.5-7 oz-eq.	7-7.5 oz-eq.	7-7.5 oz-eq.	7.5-8 oz-eq.
Milk	2-3 c.	3 c.	3 c.	3 c.	3 c.	3 c.	3 c.	3 c.
Healthy Oils	4 tsp.	5 tsp.	5 tsp.	6 tsp.	6 tsp.	7 tsp.	8 tsp.	8 tsp.

Day/Date:

Breakfast: _____ Lunch: _____

Dinner: _____ Snack: _____

Group	Fruits	Vegetables	Grains	Meat & Beans	Milk	Oils
Goal Amount						
Estimate Your Total						
Increase ⇧ or Decrease? ⇩						

Physical Activity: _____ Spiritual Activity: _____

Steps/Miles/Minutes: _____

Day/Date:

Breakfast: _____ Lunch: _____

Dinner: _____ Snack: _____

Group	Fruits	Vegetables	Grains	Meat & Beans	Milk	Oils
Goal Amount						
Estimate Your Total						
Increase ⇧ or Decrease? ⇩						

Physical Activity: _____ Spiritual Activity: _____

Steps/Miles/Minutes: _____

Day/Date:

Breakfast: _____ Lunch: _____

Dinner: _____ Snack: _____

Group	Fruits	Vegetables	Grains	Meat & Beans	Milk	Oils
Goal Amount						
Estimate Your Total						
Increase ⇧ or Decrease? ⇩						

Physical Activity: _____ Spiritual Activity: _____

Steps/Miles/Minutes: _____

Day/Date: ___

Breakfast: _____ Lunch: _____

Dinner: _____ Snack: _____
_____

Group	Fruits	Vegetables	Grains	Meat & Beans	Milk	Oils
Goal Amount						
Estimate Your Total						
Increase ⇧ or Decrease? ⇩						

Physical Activity: _____ Spiritual Activity: _____

Steps/Miles/Minutes: _____ _____

Day/Date: ___

Breakfast: _____ Lunch: _____

Dinner: _____ Snack: _____

Group	Fruits	Vegetables	Grains	Meat & Beans	Milk	Oils
Goal Amount						
Estimate Your Total						
Increase ⇧ or Decrease? ⇩						

Physical Activity: _____ Spiritual Activity: _____

Steps/Miles/Minutes: _____ _____

Day/Date: ___

Breakfast: _____ Lunch: _____

Dinner: _____ Snack: _____

Group	Fruits	Vegetables	Grains	Meat & Beans	Milk	Oils
Goal Amount						
Estimate Your Total						
Increase ⇧ or Decrease? ⇩						

Physical Activity: _____ Spiritual Activity: _____

Steps/Miles/Minutes: _____ _____

Day/Date: ___

Breakfast: _____ Lunch: _____

Dinner: _____ Snack: _____

Group	Fruits	Vegetables	Grains	Meat & Beans	Milk	Oils
Goal Amount						
Estimate Your Total						
Increase ⇧ or Decrease? ⇩						

Physical Activity: _____ Spiritual Activity: _____

Steps/Miles/Minutes: _____ _____

Live It Tracker

Name: _____ Loss/gain: _____ lbs.

Date: _____ Week #: _____ Calorie Range: _____ My food goal for next week: _____

Activity Level: None, < 30 min/day, 30-60 min/day, 60+ min/day My activity goal for next week: _____

Group	Daily Calories							
	1300-1400	1500-1600	1700-1800	1900-2000	2100-2200	2300-2400	2500-2600	2700-2800
Fruits	1.5-2 c.	1.5-2 c.	1.5-2 c.	2-2.5 c.	2-2.5 c.	2.5-3.5 c.	3.5-4.5 c.	3.5-4.5 c.
Vegetables	1.5-2 c.	2-2.5 c.	2.5-3 c.	2.5-3 c.	3-3.5 c.	3.5-4.5 c.	4.5-5 c.	4.5-5 c.
Grains	5 oz-eq.	5-6 oz-eq.	6-7 oz-eq.	6-7 oz-eq.	7-8 oz-eq.	8-9 oz-eq.	9-10 oz-eq.	10-11 oz-eq.
Meat & Beans	4 oz-eq.	5 oz-eq.	5-5.5 oz-eq.	5.5-6.5 oz-eq.	6.5-7 oz-eq.	7-7.5 oz-eq.	7-7.5 oz-eq.	7.5-8 oz-eq.
Milk	2-3 c.	3 c.	3 c.	3 c.	3 c.	3 c.	3 c.	3 c.
Healthy Oils	4 tsp.	5 tsp.	5 tsp.	6 tsp.	6 tsp.	7 tsp.	8 tsp.	8 tsp.

Day/Date: _____

Breakfast: _____ Lunch: _____

Dinner: _____ Snack: _____

Group	Fruits	Vegetables	Grains	Meat & Beans	Milk	Oils
Goal Amount						
Estimate Your Total						
Increase ⇧ or Decrease? ⇩						

Physical Activity: _____ Spiritual Activity: _____

Steps/Miles/Minutes: _____

Day/Date: _____

Breakfast: _____ Lunch: _____

Dinner: _____ Snack: _____

Group	Fruits	Vegetables	Grains	Meat & Beans	Milk	Oils
Goal Amount						
Estimate Your Total						
Increase ⇧ or Decrease? ⇩						

Physical Activity: _____ Spiritual Activity: _____

Steps/Miles/Minutes: _____

Day/Date: _____

Breakfast: _____ Lunch: _____

Dinner: _____ Snack: _____

Group	Fruits	Vegetables	Grains	Meat & Beans	Milk	Oils
Goal Amount						
Estimate Your Total						
Increase ⇧ or Decrease? ⇩						

Physical Activity: _____ Spiritual Activity: _____

Steps/Miles/Minutes: _____

Day/Date: ___

Breakfast: _____ Lunch: _____

Dinner: _____ Snack: _____
_____ _____

Group	Fruits	Vegetables	Grains	Meat & Beans	Milk	Oils
Goal Amount						
Estimate Your Total						
Increase ⬆ or Decrease? ⬇						

Physical Activity: _____ Spiritual Activity: _____

Steps/Miles/Minutes: _____ _____

Day/Date: ___

Breakfast: _____ Lunch: _____

Dinner: _____ Snack: _____
_____ _____

Group	Fruits	Vegetables	Grains	Meat & Beans	Milk	Oils
Goal Amount						
Estimate Your Total						
Increase ⬆ or Decrease? ⬇						

Physical Activity: _____ Spiritual Activity: _____

Steps/Miles/Minutes: _____ _____

Day/Date: ___

Breakfast: _____ Lunch: _____

Dinner: _____ Snack: _____
_____ _____

Group	Fruits	Vegetables	Grains	Meat & Beans	Milk	Oils
Goal Amount						
Estimate Your Total						
Increase ⬆ or Decrease? ⬇						

Physical Activity: _____ Spiritual Activity: _____

Steps/Miles/Minutes: _____ _____

Day/Date: ___

Breakfast: _____ Lunch: _____

Dinner: _____ Snack: _____
_____ _____

Group	Fruits	Vegetables	Grains	Meat & Beans	Milk	Oils
Goal Amount						
Estimate Your Total						
Increase ⬆ or Decrease? ⬇						

Physical Activity: _____ Spiritual Activity: _____

Steps/Miles/Minutes: _____ _____

let's count our miles!

Join the 100-Mile Club this Session

Can't walk that mile yet? Don't be discouraged! There are exercises you can do to strengthen your body and burn those extra calories. Keep a record on your Live It Tracker of the number of minutes you do these common physical activities, convert those minutes to miles following the chart below, and then mark off each mile you have completed on the chart found on the back of the front cover. Report your miles to your 100-Mile Club representative when you first arrive each week. Remember, you are not competing with anyone else . . . just yourself. Your job is to strive to reach 100 miles before the last meeting in this session. You can do it—just keep on moving!

Walking
slowly, 2 mph	30 min. = 156 cal. = 1 mile
moderately, 3 mph	20 min. = 156 cal. = 1 mile
very briskly, 4 mph	15 min. = 156 cal. = 1 mile
speed walking	10 min. = 156 cal. = 1 mile
up stairs	13 min. = 159 cal. = 1 mile

Running/Jogging
10 min. = 156 cal. = 1 mile

Cycling Outdoors
slowly, <10 mph	20 min. = 156 cal. = 1 mile
light effort, 10-12 mph	12 min. = 156 cal. = 1 mile
moderate effort, 12-14 mph.	10 min. = 156 cal. = 1 mile
vigorous effort, 14-16 mph	7.5 min. = 156 cal. = 1 mile
very fast, 16-19 mph	6.5 min. = 152 cal. = 1 mile

Sports Activities
Playing tennis (singles)	10 min. = 156 cal. = 1 mile
Swimming	
light to moderate effort	11 min. = 152 cal. = 1 mile
fast, vigorous effort	7.5 min. = 156 cal. = 1 mile
Softball	15 min. = 156 cal. = 1 mile
Golf	20 min. = 156 cal = 1 mile
Rollerblading	6.5 min. = 152 cal. = 1 mile
Ice skating	11 min. = 152 cal. = 1 mile

Jumping rope	7.5 min. = 156 cal. = 1 mile
Basketball	12 min. = 156 cal. = 1 mile
Soccer (casual)	15 min. = 159 cal. = 1 mile

Around the House

Mowing grass	22 min. = 156 cal. = 1 mile
Mopping, sweeping, vacuuming	19.5 min. = 155 cal. = 1 mile
Cooking	40 min. =160 cal. = 1 mile
Gardening	19 min. = 156 cal. = 1 mile
Housework (general)	35 min. = 156 cal. = 1 mile
Ironing	45 min. = 153 cal. = 1 mile
Raking leaves	25 min. = 150 cal. = 1 mile
Washing car	23 min. = 156 cal. = 1 mile
Washing dishes	45 min. = 153 cal. = 1 mile

At the Gym

Stair machine	8.5 min. = 155 cal. = 1 mile
Stationary bike	
slowly, 10 mph	30 min. = 156 cal. = 1 mile
moderately, 10-13 mph	15 min. = 156 cal. = 1 mile
vigorously, 13-16 mph	7.5 min. = 156 cal. = 1 mile
briskly, 16-19 mph	6.5 min. = 156 cal. = 1 mile
Elliptical trainer	12 min. = 156 cal. = 1 mile
Weight machines (used vigorously)	13 min. = 152 cal.=1 mile
Aerobics	
low impact	15 min. = 156 cal. = 1 mile
high impact	12 min. = 156 cal. = 1 mile
water	20 min. = 156 cal. = 1 mile
Pilates	15 min. = 156 cal. = 1 mile
Raquetball (casual)	15 min. = 159 cal. = 1 mile
Stretching exercises	25 min. = 150 cal. = 1 mile
Weight lifting (also works for weight machines used moderately or gently)	30 min. = 156 cal. = 1 mile

Family Leisure

Playing piano	37 min. = 155 cal. = 1 mile
Jumping rope	10 min. = 152 cal. = 1 mile
Skating (moderate)	20 min. = 152 cal. = 1 mile
Swimming	
moderate	17 min. = 156 cal. = 1 mile
vigorous	10 min. = 148 cal. = 1 mile
Table tennis	25 min. = 150 cal. = 1 mile
Walk/run/play with kids	25 min. = 150 cal. = 1 mile

Week 2: Growing in Love

But God demonstrates his own love for us in this: While we were still sinners, Christ died for us.

Week 3: Growing in Hope

"For I know the plans I have for you," declares the Lord, "plans to prosper you and not to harm you, plans to give you hope and a future."

Growing in the Fruit of the Spirit

Growing in the Fruit of the Spirit
Scripture Memory Verses:

ROMANS 5:8
JEREMIAH 29:11
HEBREWS 11:6
GALATIANS 5:22-23
NEHEMIAH 8:10

PHILIPPIANS 4:7
GALATIANS 6:9
COLOSSIANS 3:12
MATTHEW 11:29
GALATIANS 5:16

How to Use These Cards:

Separate cards from the Bible study book. These cards are designed to be used when exercising. To do this, you may want to punch a hole in the upper left corner of the cards and place on a ring. When you have finished memorizing all the verses from one study, add the new Bible study cards to the ring and continue practicing the old verses while learning the new ones. Cards may be placed anywhere you will see them regularly—on the dashboard of your car, on a mirror, on a desk. After you have memorized the verse, begin using the reverse side of the card so the reference is connected to the verse. This is a great way to practice the verses you have already learned.

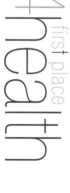

first place
4health
discover a new way to healthy living

ROMANS 5:8

JEREMIAH 29:11

Week 4: Growing in Faith

And without faith it is impossible to please God, because anyone who comes to him must believe that he exists and that he rewards those who earnestly seek him.

Week 5: Growing in Goodness

But the fruit of the Spirit is love, joy, peace, patience, kindness, goodness, faithfulness, gentleness and self-control. Against such things there is no law.

Week 6: Growing in Joy

Do not grieve, for the joy of the LORD is your strength.

Week 7: Growing in Peace

And the peace of God, which transcends all understanding, will guard your hearts and your minds in Christ Jesus.

NEHEMIAH 8:10

HEBREWS 11:6

PHILIPPIANS 4:7

GALATIANS 5:22-23